Nursing Quality Measurement:

A Review of Nursing Studies 1995–2000

Marilyn J. Rantz, PhD, RN, FAAN
Jane E. Bostick, PhD, RN
C. Jo Riggs, MSN, RN

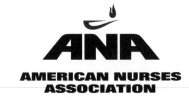

ANA
AMERICAN NURSES ASSOCIATION
WASHINGTON, D.C.

Library of Congress Cataloging-in-Publication Data

Rantz, Marilyn J.
Nursing quality measurement : a review of nursing studies 1995–2000 / Marilyn J. Rantz,
Jane E. Bostick, C. Jo Riggs.
       p. ; cm.
   Includes bibliographical references.
   ISBN 1-55810-201-9
1. Nursing—Quality control.   2. Nursing—Standards.   3. Outcome assessment (Medical
care)   I. Bostick, Jane E.   II. Riggs, C. Jo.   III. American Nurses Association.   IV. Title.
[DNLM: 1. Nursing Care—standards—United States—Abstracts.   2. Evaluation Studies —
United States—Abstracts.   3. Outcome and Process Assessment (Health Care)—United
States—Abstracts.   4. Quality Assurance, Health Care—standards—United States—Abstracts.
ZWY 100 R213n 2002]
RT85.5.R362   2002
362.1′73′0685—dc21   2002014075

Published by
American Nurses Publishing
600 Maryland Avenue, SW
Suite 100 West
Washington, D.C. 20024-2571

ISBN 1-55810-201-9

NQM22   1.5M   09/02

Contents

Using This Book

Quality-related terminology, categories of the studies, review methodology, and conclusions and recommendations of the reviews are discussed in Chapter 1. Appendix A lists the reference works that underlie those discussions in Chapter 1 and each chapter's overview, while Appendix C indexes all the studies that we have reviewed. The glossary of Appendix B lists all the acronyms used in this book.

While the topics within each chapter, listed in the table of contents and the index, are the most obvious points of access to the book's contents, we have provided another: the following tables will direct you to studies that deal with some clinical topics in pediatric, women's health, geriatric, and adult health nursing care.

Pediatrics topics	See these pages
Anemia	20–21
Catheters	88–89
Child health	22–23
CVP (central venous pressure) occlusion	87
Infections	75
Immunizations	20
Pain management	57–58
Skin integrity	56

Women's health topics	See these pages:
Breast cancer	94
Breastfeeding	81
Contraception	16–17
Neonatal care	68, 101
Postpartum care	23, 35–36, 52, 80, 95
Pregnancy	12, 13

Geriatrics	See these pages
Alzheimer's	120, 133
Bathing	120–21, 123
Constipation, bowels	117
Depression	27, 77, 127, 139
Dementia, confusion	83, 119, 127, 129, 132–33, 134, 139
Diabetes	139
End of life care	134–35, 139
Falls and injuries	42, 109, 119
Functional status	27, 80, 123
Incontinence	80, 121
Infections	121, 132
Medication compliance	27–28
Pain management	57–58, 139
Physical restraint	115–16, 120, 123
Pressure ulcers	42, 44, 114–15
Psychiatric and psychosocial	103, 118, 119, 120, 122, 123, 128
Rheumatiod arthritis	16
Skin care	120–21
Weight, nutrition, meals	117, 118, 122, 139

Adult health topic	See these pages:
Alcohol-related diagnoses	110
Cancer/oncology	43, 57, 94, 98
Cardiopulmonary (general)	21, 43, 46, 70, 77, 87–88
CABG (coronary artery bypass graft)/atrial fibrillation	50, 52, 77
CHF (congestive heart failure)	70, 78, 82
Confusion	84
Constipation and bowels	12, 79
COPD (chronic obstructive pulmonary disease)	42
Cystitis	13
Diabetes	11, 15–16, 34–35, 47–48, 83–84
Dialysis	11
End of life care	96, 103, 140
Falls and injuries	43, 44–45, 46, 54, 61, 62, 110
Heart attacks/MI (myocardial infarction)	40–41, 42, 70, 79, 80, 81–82, 85
HIV/AIDS	14, 29–30, 89, 139
Infections	43, 44–45, 46, 62, 73, 75
Kidney disease	47–48, 78–79
Medication errors	43, 44–45, 54, 62, 65
Mortality	11, 41, 44–45, 53
Nutrition	35
Pain management	42, 57, 58–60
Physical restraint	55, 56
Pneumonia	70, 73–75
Pressure ulcers	44–45, 54–55
Psychiatric and psychosocial	50–51, 86, 89, 92, 98–99
Rheumatoid arthritis	16
Seizures	88
Spinal injuries	88
Stroke	78, 140, 141
Surgery	59, 70, 76, 77, 80, 82, 84, 95
Surgery (post-op)	76, 80, 106, 138

continued

Adult health topic	See these pages:
Transplant and replacement surgery	78–79
THR/TKR (total hip replacement/total knee replacement)	78, 84–85, 86
Tuberculosis	73–74
Trauma, emergency room situations	48, 53, 94, 95, 101, 104
Vascular/venous access issues	46, 86–87, 88–89, 119
Vital signs	87–88

Overview of Nursing Quality Measurement | 1

During the past 20 years, the American Nurses' Association has commissioned three reviews of nursing quality measurement. Any review of quality requires a clear understanding of the terminology used to measure this multi-faceted concept. Definitions of quality, standards, and related terminology are discussed, setting the stage for the review of nursing quality measurement literature. The literature is summarized for the years 1995–2000 and recommendations are set forth for nursing action. Our final recommendation captures the essence of this review: nursing can and should provide leadership in quality improvement for health care. Nurses have a long and strong history of quality and measurement research that can be invaluable to the outcomes of patients and collaboration with other health care providers.

Quality, Standards, and Related Terminology

Most definitions of quality in the nursing literature are exact quotes or slight variations of the definition put forth by the Joint Commission on Accreditation of Healthcare Organizations (JCAHO):

> Quality of patient care is defined as the degree to which patient care services increase the probability of desired patient outcomes and reduce the probability of undesired outcomes, given the current state of knowledge. (Accreditation Manual for Hospitals 1990, 310).

The Institute of Medicine's definition is very similar:

> Quality of care is the degree to which health services for individuals and populations increase the likelihood of desired health outcomes and are consistent with current professional knowledge. (Harris-Wehling 1990, 128).

In 1993, JCAHO expanded its definition to include potential components of quality: "accessibility of care, appropriateness of care, continuity of care, effectiveness of care, efficacy of care, efficiency of care, patient perspective issues, safety of the care environment, and timeliness of care" (Accreditation Manual for Hospitals, 1993, 234).

These definitions have remained consistent in the 1990s with slight variations. Most recently, an Institute of Medicine Committee proposed six aims for improvement of the health care delivery system. They proposed that health care should be safe, effective, patient-centered, timely, efficient, and equitable (Committee on Quality of Care in America, 2001).

Katz and Green (1997) believe that a universal definition of quality is not forthcoming, but that standards define quality. In their opinion, the quality of care that is expected from a health care facility is made explicit by written standards that direct the way services are to be provided. Standards define a set of rules, actions, or conditions. Rules relate to the structure of the service, actions to the process of how the service is delivered, and conditions to the results or outcomes of the service (Katz & Green, 1997). The terms *structure, process,* and *outcome standards* have been pervasive in nursing literature for more than three decades. They are derived from the work of Donabedian and from the quality assurance (QA) model developed by the American Nurses Association and widely disseminated in the 1970s.

In the early 1990s, the term *standard* took on a broader meaning as "an authoritative statement enumerated and promulgated by the profession by which the quality of practice, service, or education can be judged" (American Nurses Association, 1991, 7). The term is differentiated from standards of nursing practice, standards of care, and standards of professional performance. Standards of nursing practice are "an authoritative statement that describes a level of performance common to the profession of nursing by which the quality of nursing practice can be judged" (American Nurses Association, 1991, 7). Standards of nursing practice include both standards of care and standards of professional performance. Standards of care describe a "competent level of care demonstrated by a process of accurate assessment and diagnosis, planning, appropriate interventions, and predicted patient outcomes" (American Nurses Association, 1991, 8). The American Nurses Association (ANA) has also defined guidelines, universal practice guidelines, specialty practice guidelines, criteria, and procedures. *Criteria* are variables known to be relevant, measurable indicators of the standards of practice. *Procedures* describe recommended actions for the completion of a specified task or function. These actions may be specific to an institution or applicable across settings (American Nurses Association, 1991, 8).

Quality cannot be measured until it is defined and outcomes are specified (Gardner, 1992). But the issue of specifying nursing outcomes is controversial. Marek (1989 defined outcome as a measurable change in a client's health status related to the receipt of nursing care. Clearly, this definition focuses on *nursing* outcomes. According to Hegyvary (1991), however, the term *nursing outcome* should rarely (if ever) be used because outcome is a patient response to care, not a provider response.

The National Center for Nursing Research (NCNR) initiated a major effort regarding outcomes in May 1990 when it convened an expert planning group to discuss patient outcomes and nursing research (Johnson & McCloskey, 1992). This group coined the term *nurse-sensitive outcomes*, referring to patient outcomes that are sensitive to nursing intervention. Major research at the University of Iowa focuses on identifying and testing nurse-sensitive outcomes (Johnson, et al., 2001; Johnson, Maas, & Moorhead, 2000; McCloskey & Bulechek, 2000).

JCAHO has stimulated much change in quality measurement over the past three decades. The terms *quality assurance, quality assessment, continuous quality improvement, total quality management, quality improvement, performance improvement,* or *organizational performance improvement* have been promoted by JCAHO and others and attempt to capture the essence of quality measurement activities (Joint Commission, 1998). These words have dual meanings: they describe the effort to measure the quality of care delivered within health care organizations, as well as the effort to measure the quality of care delivered within health care organizations, as well as the effort to analyze the results of those measurements and ensure that future actions will result in targeted patient outcomes. In other words, the terms attempt to describe a process of quality measurement. This process assumes, and in fact requires, that appropriate systems be in place within health care organizations to collect data and ensure that corrective actions are taken when necessary. Performance improvement attempts to capture the essence of constantly evaluating the performance of health care providers while upgrading or improving services.

A framework for a National Health Care Quality Report has been proposed that is a matrix of components of health care quality (safety, effectiveness, patient centeredness, timeliness) and consumer perspectives on health care needs (staying healthy, getting better, living with illness or disability, and coping with end of life) (Committee on the National Quality Report on Health Care Delivery, 2001). This framework has the potential to involve the consumer as an active, rather than passive, participant in health care quality. It will be interesting to follow the implementation of such a quality perspective. Although the terminology may shift, the fundamentals of describing measurable quality criteria, measuring performance against these criteria, and setting actions in place to improve performance remain the same. A key point that has stood the test of time is that changes in nursing practice based on quality measurement activities require formal action strategies to stabilize innovations within health care organizations (Miller & Rantz, 1989). Organizational structures and support systems must be in place to ensure optimal integration of quality measurement findings into actual clinical practice.

Review of Literature

To ensure an inclusive investigation of quality measurement materials produced during the last 5 years, the researchers used two methods to review the nursing literature. These methods are consistent with a previous approach used by the first author to review nursing quality measurement studies (Rantz, 1995).

First, an electronic computer database (CINAHL) was searched for articles published between 1995 and 2000 that used the terms quality monitoring, quality of care research, quality of health care, quality assurance, quality assessment, or quality in the title or abstract. Other terms used in the search strategies were clinical indicators, quality of nursing care, quality circles, quality control, quality improvement, quality management, and quality assessment. The electronic search yielded 4,898 citations. This set of citations was then limited to research, journal articles, nursing journals, and United States journals resulting in a narrowed set of 388 citations. A manual review of citations and abstracts was performed to eliminate those articles without a clear research focus. Inclusion criteria for the manual review included either

- a focus on nursing,
- a description of the potential impact or measure of some aspects of nursing care, or
- nurses listed as authors.

A total of 157 articles were eliminated, leaving 231 articles identified in the electronic search.

In the second method, the researchers conducted a hand search of the following journals published between 1995 and 2000:

- Joint Commission Journal on Quality Improvement
- Journal for Healthcare Quality
- Journal of Nursing Scholarship *(formerly* IMAGE: Journal of Nursing Scholarship*)*
- Journal of Gerontological Nursing
- Journal of Nursing Administration
- Journal of Nursing Care Quality
- Nursing Administration Quarterly
- Nursing Management
- The Gerontologist

Articles authored by nurses or teams involving nurses and describing efforts to define or measure quality were abstracted. A total of 89 articles were identified from the hand search. This review of nursing studies revealed 322 citations ($n = 315$ studies and 7 discussion/process articles). The 1995–2000 review had twice the number of studies identified than found in the 1989–1994 study ($n = 135$ studies and a sample of discussion/process articles [$n = 23$] for a total of 158 citations).

Using both approaches, the researchers identified and abstracted 322 articles and carefully reviewed and categorized them according to setting and major focus (Table 1-1). For the sake of consistency, the specified practice settings are categorized in the same way as the first review (1995). These categories include hospital-based, home health care, long-term care, ambulatory care, and community health studies, as well as studies that cross all settings. All are research articles except for seven nursing discussion/process articles, which are included

T A B L E 1 - 1 Reviewed and Abstracted NQM Studies by Practice Setting and Major Focus

Topics	Number of Studies
Ambulatory Care Nursing Quality Measurement Studies (N = 21)	
Quality outcomes/attributes	2
Quality improvement projects	6
Practice guidelines	2
Patient satisfaction	3
Instruments	2
Patient education	2
Health maintenance organizations (HMO)	3
Nursing center	1
Community Health Nursing Quality Measurement Studies (N = 10)	
Quality outcomes	7
Program evaluation	3
Home Health Nursing Quality Measurement Studies (N = 27)	
Quality outcomes/quality improvement	8
Patient satisfaction/staff perceptions	6
Program evaluation/regulatory	4
Documentation/OASIS	4
Discharge planning/patient teaching	2
Case management/critical paths	2
Instruments	1
Hospital-Based Nursing Quality Measurement Studies (N = 179)	
Quality outcome measures	16
Methods of quality measurement	7
Case management/clinical pathways	13
Patient safety	9
Pain and pain management	12
Care delivery models	9
Staff and staffing	10
Organizational restructuring/redesign	11
Infection control	7
Specific clinical issues	28
Clinical issues related to care processes	10
Work environment	8
Patient and staff perceptions of quality	20
Patient/caregiver satisfaction	15
Technology use	3
Patient education	1

TABLE 1-1 (*continued*)

Topics	Number of Studies
Veterans Affairs Nursing Quality Measurement Studies (*N* = 5)	
Clinical issues	3
Quality improvement	2
Long-Term Care Nursing Quality Measurement Studies (*N* = 55)	
Clinical issues	21
Quality measurement	9
Staffing	8
MDS/quality indicators	8
Satisfaction with care	5
Family involvement	2
End of life	2
Nursing Quality Measurement Studies That Cross All Settings (*N* – 18)	
Quality improvement	6
Clinical issues	6
Managed care	4
Satisfaction with care	2

T A B L E 1 - 2   Sample of Discussion/Process Articles About Quality Measurement and Nurse-Sensitive Outcomes (Not reports of studies) (*N* = 7)

Topics	Number of Studies
Nursing outcomes classification (NOC)	4
Quality measurement and research priorities	2
Nursing intervention classification (NIC)	1

due to their significance to the topic of nursing quality measurement and nurse-sensitive outcomes (Table 1-2). Chapters 2 through 8 include abstracts of the nursing quality measurement studies, and Chapter 9 includes the sample of discussion/process articles. Each citation is listed alphabetically by author in Appendix C.

Conclusion and Recommendations

This is the third literature review about nursing's contribution to quality measurement in health care. Each review has examined the literature for a period of 5 or 10 years. The first was focused on the care of older people and located 345 research studies reported in the nursing literature from 1980 to 1990 (Lang, Kraegel, Rantz, & Krejci, 1990). The second identified 135 nursing studies and a sample of 23 discussion/process articles focused on a broad range of quality of care issues for 5 years, 1989 to 1994 (Rantz, 1995). This third review has revealed 315 nursing studies and a small sample of 7 discussion/process articles focused on quality of care for the years 1995 to 2000. It is clear that nursing researchers are contributing to the evaluation of quality of care in America.

The recommendations based on the second review are remarkably stable and relevant based on this latest review. As we move into the twenty-first century, it is now imperative that nursing take the lead in ensuring that critical data are collected in computerized medical record, billing, federal, state, and other data bases. These critical elements include a unique identifier for each nurse so that the provider of care can be linked to patient outcomes; outcomes of patients that can reflect the impact of nursing care provided or not provided; standardized language for identifying patient problems and interventions that nurses use to help patients and other health care providers manage those problems; and data about staffing and staff mix of nursing and other direct care providers in all health care settings.

Similar to the 1995 recommendations, the following are made based on the review of nursing quality measurement studies in health care for the years 1995 to 2000:

1. Incorporate the NMDS elements into all computerized medical record systems and into federal and state data bases as they are revised. Collecting these elements should be viewed as essential data as regulations are promulgated to enforce legislation written to ensure quality of health care services.
2. Document nursing hours of care per patient, educational preparation of the nurse provider, and the use of assistive personnel in the delivery of care. Each nurse should have a unique provider identifier. Care delivery hours should be included in all large data sets for all settings.
3. A system for determining what constitutes appropriate outcomes for patients in different settings is needed. Data elements for these outcome measures must be included in large data sets for all settings. The system must be sensitive to an individual's potential for self-care or recovery.
4. Continued support for research efforts to identify nurse-sensitive outcomes and the relationship among nursing diagnoses, interventions, outcomes, staffing, and staff mix is essential. Support of standardization so that these elements are included in large data sets is also essential.
5. Nursing can and should provide leadership in quality improvement for health care. Nurses have a long and strong history of quality measurement research that can be invaluable to the outcomes of patients and collaboration with other health care providers.

Ambulatory Care Nursing Quality Measurement Studies | 2

Overview

As with other settings, there was a noticeable increase in the number of studies (21 in this review compared to 9 in Rantz, 1995) focusing on quality in diverse ambulatory care settings, including health maintenance organizations (Banks, Palmer, Berwick, & Plsek, 1995; Hoare, Lacoste, Haro, & Conyers, 1999), an academic nursing center (Adams et al., 1996), and various out-patient clinics. Attributes of quality were identified from a consumer perspective (Oermann, Dillon, & Templin, 2000; Oermann & Templin, 2000). Consumer satisfaction and perception were the most commonly measured indicators of quality. Three studies in this review examined customer satisfaction with primary care services provided by nurse-practitioners (Cole, Mackey, & Lindenberg, 1999; Langner & Hutelmyer, 1995; Larrabee, Ferri, & Hartig, 1997). As nurse-practitioner's scope of practice continues to expand, additional studies will be necessary to evaluate their effectiveness.

In addition to customer satisfaction, a variety of other quality measurements were found in the ambulatory care setting. These measures were tailored to each study site and to a specific patient population. Quality measures included patient screening rates for diabetic retinopathy (Buonaccoro, 1999), proficiency of diabetic self-monitoring of blood glucose (Bergenstal et al., 2000), and outcomes of prenatal care (Lowry & Beikirich, 1998). Staff surveys were used to collect data regarding practice changes in dialysis units (Frederick, Frankenfield, Biddle, & Sims, 1995) and to evaluate a high-risk pregnancy program (Mackey & Sobral, 1997).

The diversity of settings and outcome measures make it difficult to draw conclusions from this group of studies. Customer satisfaction is an important measure of quality across ambulatory care settings. Different patient satisfaction instruments were used in each of the studies reviewed, making generalization of findings difficult. Instruments have been developed and tested to measure patient satisfaction with nursing care (Forbes and Brown, 1995) and with care by nurse-practitioners (Cole, Mackey, & Lindenberg, 1999). The use of these and other established instruments would make findings more consistent across settings. Consistent definition and measurement of other quality measures across ambulatory care settings would also make the collection of aggregate data possible, and make it possible to compare quality measurement within and across systems.

The 21 ambulatory care nursing quality measurement studies in this chapter are organized as follows:

▌ Quality outcomes/attributes
▌ Quality improvement programs and projects
▌ Practice guidelines
▌ Patient satisfaction
▌ Instruments
▌ Patient education
▌ Health maintenance organizations (HMOs)
▌ Nursing center

Quality Outcomes/Attributes (N = 2)

Author(s): Oermann, M. H., Dillon, S. L., & Templin, T.
Article Title: Indicators of quality of care in clinics: patients' perspectives
Journal Title: Journal for Healthcare Quality
Volume (Issue): 22(6) **Year:** 2000 (November–December) **Pages:** 9–12

Summary: The purpose of this exploratory study was to identify indicators of quality of health care and nursing care that were important to patients ($N = 119$) of a large Midwestern urban ambulatory care facility. The most important indicators of health care quality identified were getting better, getting care and services when needed, and having diagnoses and treatment options explained. The most important indicators of nursing care quality were communicating with the nurse, being treated with respect, being cared for by nurses who were up to date, teaching by the nurse, and not being rushed through the visit.

Author(s): Oermann, M. H., & Templin, T.
Article Title: Important attributes of quality health care: Consumer perspectives
Journal Title: *Journal of Nursing Scholarship*
Volume (Issue): 32(2) **Year:** 2000 **Pages:** 167–172

Summary: The purposes of this exploratory study were to (a) identify the importance to consumers of attributes of health care quality and nursing care quality, and (b) examine the relationship of consumer perspectives to health status and selected demographic variables. Consumers ($N = 239$) were recruited from waiting rooms of clinics and in neighborhoods of a large metropolitan area in the Midwestern United States that included both urban and suburban populations. Study instruments included the Quality Health Care Questionnaire (QHCQ) and the SF-36 Health Survey. The most important indicators of high-quality nursing care were (a) being cared for by nurses who are up to date and well informed; (b) being able to communicate with the nurse; (c) spending enough time with the nurse and not feeling rushed during the visit; (d) having a nurse teach about the illness, medications, treatments, and staying healthy; and (e)being able to call a nurse with questions. The lowest-rated item was having an opportunity to be cared for by nurse-practitioners. Ratings differed by race, age, years of education, income, and health status. The importance that consumers place on teaching by the nurse was emphasized, particularly among people with less education, low income levels, and chronic illnesses.

Quality Improvement Programs and Projects (N = 6)

Author(s): Buonaccoro, K. M.
Article Title: Diabetic retinopathy screening: A clinical quality improvement project
Journal Title: *Journal for Healthcare Quality*
Volume (Issue): 21(6): **Year:** 1999 **Pages:** 35–38

Summary: This article describes a quality improvement project to improve diabetic retinopathy screening rates of BlueCross/BlueShield members in the Rochester area. A quality improvement team was formed that included a physician, registered nurses, a data analyst, and a health educator. Using HEDIS data, the rate of annual eye examinations was for diabetic patients improved from 42.7% in 1995 to 54.2% in 1996, and 58.1% in 1997. Over this period, 2,295 additional members of the health plan with diabetes received eye examinations.

Author(s): Frederick, P. R., Frankenfield, D. L., Biddle, M. G., & Sims, T. W.
Article Title: Changes in dialysis units' quality improvement practices from 1994 to 1996.
Journal Title: *ANNA Journal*
Volume (Issue): 25(5) **Year:** 1998 (October) **Pages:** 469–478

Summary: In 1994, the Health Care Financing Administration (HCFA) initiated a nationwide effort to improve care to Medicare's end-stage renal disease (ESRD) beneficiaries by reshaping the manner in which the ESRD Network Organizations measure and assess the quality of dialysis services. The new approach was named the ESRD Health Care Quality Improvement Program (HCQIP). In an effort to document changes in dialysis quality practices associated with the ESRD HCQIP, surveys were sent by network staff to the head nurses of all dialysis units in 1994, and a random sample of units in 1996. Analysis of the survey responses was performed identifying self-reported changes in dialysis units' quality improvement activities. Results indicate that practice changes are taking place, that they are generalizable to all dialysis units in the country, and that they are associated with improvement in patient outcomes. Trends in quality improvement activities are identified and conclusions are drawn about what impact these activities have on patient care.

Author(s): Hearn, K., Dailey, M., Harris M. T., & Bodian, C.
Article Title: Reduce costs and improve patient satisfaction with home pre-operative bowel preparations
Journal Title: *Nursing Case Management*
Volume (Issue): 5(1)   Year: 2000 (January–February)   Pages: 13–25

Summary: The results of a home-based, preoperative bowel preparation, with and without the support of home care services, are compared with hospital-based preoperative bowel preparation. Length of stay, morbidity and mortality rates, issues of patient satisfaction, and demographics are reported. The method and tools used in planning, implementing, and evaluating the home preoperative bowel preparation program are also shared. Other issues discussed are the health care market forces that promote an increased value of care; economic and patient satisfaction considerations by employers, payers, and patients; the increasing influence of patient choice on health care provider selection and care setting preferences; the nursing workforce issues related to the impending shortage; and issues of regulatory and accrediting agencies.

Author(s): Horowitz, C. R., Goldberg, H. I., Martin, D. P., Wagner, E. H., Fihn, S. D., Christensen, D. B., & Cheadle, A. D.
Article Title: Conducting a randomized controlled trial of CQI and academic detailing to implement clinical guidelines
Journal Title: *Journal on Quality Improvement*
Volume (Issue): 22(11)   Year: 1996   Pages: 734–750

Summary: Given the growing interest in vigorous evaluation of multifaceted quality improvement programs, this article is offered as an example of the organization, methodology, and implementation of just such a program.

Author(s): Lowry, L. W. & Beikirch, P.
Article Title: Effect of comprehensive care on pregnancy outcomes... Ambulatory health care center for women and children called Genesis
Journal Title: *Applied Nursing Research*
Volume (Issue): 11(2)   Year: 1998 (May)   Pages: 55–61

Summary: The purpose of the study was to compare pregnancy outcomes of low socioeconomic pregnant women receiving prenatal care at a prototype, comprehensive, multidisciplinary tertiary care clinic with outcomes of a matched sample who received prenatal care from a variety of area public health clinics. Multidisciplinary clinic subjects were matched by age, race, and parity to 175 control subjects selected from labor and delivery logs of the general hospital that services the entire community. There were significant differences between groups on the measures of gestational age ($t[174] = 2.50, p < .01$), maternal risk factors ($t[174] = 11.12, p < .0$), and infant complications ($t[174] = 5.86, p < .01$). Infant birthweight and APGAR scores were not significantly different between the multidisciplinary clinic subjects and the matched sample. This study showed the importance of comprehensive prenatal care for low socioeconomic women at high risk for obstetrical and medical complications.

Author(s): Mackey, M. C., & Sobral, M.
Article Title: Staff evaluation of a high-risk pregnancy program
Journal Title: *Public Health Nursing*
Volume (Issue): 14(2)   Year: 1997 (April)   Pages: 101–110

Summary: The purpose of this study was to obtain the staff's evaluation of this high-risk pregnancy program. Clinical, supervisory, and clerical staff ($N = 182$) completed a questionnaire about the operation of the program and its perceived benefits. Staff identified program strengths: nurse case management, interdisciplinary structure, quality care, and positive health outcomes. Staff also identified program limitations, including limited staff and time, inflexible protocols, administrative tasks, and narrow enrollment criteria. The majority of staff reported that the following barriers interfered with the effective operation of the program: paperwork, limited support, time, difficulty locating patients, and mandated time frames for patient contact. The majority of staff also reported that transportation most interfered with patient access to the program. The findings of this study support the need for ongoing staff evaluation of all perinatal health care programs.

Practice Guidelines (N = 2)

Author(s): Goode, C. J., Tanaka, D. J., Krugman, M., O'Connor, P. A., Bailey P., Deutchman, M., & Stolpman, N. M.
Article Title: Outcomes from use of an evidence-based practice guideline
Journal Title: *Nursing Economics*
Volume (Issue): 18(4)   Year: 2000 (July–August)   Pages: 202–207

Summary: The purpose of this project was to generate a practice guideline for the treatment of uncomplicated acute cystitis in a female population, to determine the extent to which the guideline would be used by providers, and to measure the cost and quality of outcomes from its use. A retrospective chart review was used to gather pre-guideline practice and cost data. Measurements included the type, frequency, and duration of antibiotic therapy and the use of urine cultures and both complications and routine follow-up visits. The implementation of an outpatient practice guideline resulted in a significant change in antibiotic prescribing and a trend toward a change in ordering cultures and clinic follow-up.

Author(s): Gruber, J. L.
Article Title: Strategies for implementing quantifiable group practice guidelines
Journal Title: *Journal for Healthcare Quality*
Volume (Issue): 21(4)   Year: 1999   Pages: 11–20

Summary: Physician project teams were developed for the purpose of the development of best-practice guidelines for seven selected topics. Scannable audit tools were developed using Teleform software, and peer chart audits were done. Data were also collected through disease-specific patient surveys. Each guideline was pilot tested for 3 months. Revised guidelines were then distributed to providers for review. The author reports that outcome measurements are planned.

Patient Satisfaction (N = 3)

Author(s): Langner, S. R. & Hutelmyer, C.
Article Title: Patient satisfaction with outpatient human immunodeficiency virus care as delivered by nurse practitioners and physicians
Journal Title: *Holistic Nursing Practice*
Volume (Issue): 10(1) **Year:** 1995 **Pages:** 54–60

Summary: Primary care of patients infected with human immunodeficiency virus (HIV) present major challenges for the nurse-practitioner. A patient satisfaction survey designed to include aspects of care specific to HIV was given to HIV-positive individuals presenting for care at an urban medical teaching clinic. Fifty-two patients with HIV/acquired immunodeficiency syndrome (AIDS) completed the patient satisfaction survey between February and May of 1994. Overall satisfaction with patient care was high. When nurse-practitioners were compared with physician providers, nurse-practitioners fared more favorably in the areas relating to clinic waiting time, provider knowledge about the disease, continuity of care, and patient education.

Author(s): Larrabee, J. H., Ferri, J. A., & Hartig, M. T.
Article Title: Patient satisfaction with nurse practitioner care in primary care
Journal Title: *Journal of Nursing Care Quality*
Volume (Issue): 11(5) **Year:** 1997 (June) **Pages:** 9–14

Summary: This quantitative, descriptive pilot study assessed patient satisfaction with care provided by four nurse-practitioners using a modified version of the Di Tomasso-Willard Patient Satisfaction Questionnaire. Results indicated high satisfaction with care in all groups, but there were differences among the groups on 26% of the items and on three of the five subscales. The implication is that nurse-practitioners need to identify and improve those differences of care for which patients are less satisfied.

Author(s): Morishita, L., Boult, C., Boult, L., Smith, S., & Pacala, J. T.
Article Title: Satisfaction with outpatient geriatric evaluation and management (GEM)
Journal Title: *Gerontologist*
Volume (Issue): 38(3) **Year:** 1998 **Pages:** 303–308

Summary: The purpose of this study was to evaluate high-risk older adults' satisfaction with outpatient geriatric evaluation and management (GEM). Community-dwelling Medicare beneficiaries ($n = 522$) age 70 years and older who had a high probability of repeated admission to hospitals ($p_{ra} > .40$) were randomly assigned to receive either usual care or GEM for 6 months. Despite the stresses imposed by outpatient GEM (eg, new relationships with providers, frequent office visits, and changes in treatments), the mean satisfaction scores of the recipients of GEM were 9% higher than those of the recipients of usual care (4.31 versus 3.96, $p < .001$). The primary physicians of GEM recipients were also highly satisfied with GEM care.

Instruments (N = 2)

Author(s): Cole, F. L., Mackey, T., & Lindenberg, J.
Article Title: Search and research. Quality improvement: Psychometric evaluation of patient satisfaction with nurse practitioner care instrument
Journal Title: *Journal of the American Academy of Nurse Practitioners*
Volume (Issue): 11(11)   **Year:** 1999 (November)   **Pages:** 471–475

Summary: The purpose of this project was to assess the psychometric properties of an instrument used to measure satisfaction with care provide by nurse-practitioners. The 31-item instrument was constructed through a review of the literature and through examination of extant instruments. Of the 387 questionnaires distributed, 182 were returned for a response rate of 47%. The initial psychometric assessment provides support for reliability (internal consistency) and validity of this instrument.

Author(s): Forbes, M. L., & Brown, H. N.
Article Title: Developing an instrument for measuring patient satisfaction
Journal Title: *AORN Journal*
Volume (Issue): 61(4):   **Year:** 1995   **Pages:** 737, 739, 741–743

Summary: We developed a 21-item questionnaire to evaluate the effectiveness of nursing care provided in an outpatient surgery center. The four constructs of the instrument for measuring patient satisfaction are caring, continuity of care, competence of nurses, and education of patients and family members. Content validity and test–retest reliability have been established. Using this tool to analyze patients' responses to nursing care can help perioperative nurses improve patient care and patient satisfaction.

Patient Education (N = 3)

Author(s): Bergenstal, R., Pearson, J., Cembrowski, G. S., Bina, D., Davidson J., & List, S.
Article Title: Identifying variables associated with inaccurate self-monitoring of blood glucose: Proposed guidelines to improve accuracy
Journal Title: *Diabetes Educator*
Volume (Issue): 26(6)   **Year:** 2000 (November–December)   **Pages:** 981–989

Summary: This study was conducted to evaluate patients' proficiency in self-monitoring of blood glucose (SMBG). Diabetes nurse educators in four suburban Minneapolis clinic sites surveyed the SMBG training/cure practices of 280 patients with type 1 and type 2 diabetes. Of the 280 participants, 19% had blood glucose test results greater than the 15% limit for meter accuracy. After reeducation, 69% of those who had initially failed achieved acceptable results. The most significant problems were lack of periodic meter technique evaluation, difficulty using wipe meters, incorrect use of control solutions, lack of hand washing even when observed, and unclean meters. As a result of the study, guidelines were subsequently developed to evaluate meter accuracy in an outpatient setting. Further effort is needed to establish standards for evaluating SMBG.

Author(s): Burma, M. R., Rachow, J. W., Kolluri, S., & Saag, K. G.
Article Title: Methotrexate patient education: A quality improvement study
Journal Title: *Arthritis Care & Research*
Volume (Issue): 9(3)   **Year:** 1996 (June)   **Pages:** 216–222

Summary: To determine patients' knowledge of the safe use and toxicity of methotrexate (MTX) and to define educational interventions implemented by a rheumatology nurse that improved patients' understanding of MTX therapy. One hundred eighty-three patients from a university-based rheumatology clinic who were taking MTX completed an initial knowledge questionnaire concerning the proper use and possible toxicity of MTX. Following completion, a nurse reviewed the correct answers with each patient and provided written information on MTX. One hundred thirty-eight of these patients completed a follow-up questionnaire at the next visit or by mail. The questionnaires were analyzed, and a total MTX knowledge score was calculated. MTX knowledge improved significantly between questionnaires. After accounting for a person's initial questionnaire score, the addition of a supplemental "MTX pocket-card" was associated with a higher score on the follow-up. Patients over age 55 were four times more likely to have a poorer score compared with patients under age 45. Knowledge of the toxicity and safe use of MTX was significantly improved by a patient education program utilizing a rheumatology nurse. Older individuals appear to be at higher risk for knowledge deficits. A supplemental MTX pocket-card proved to be a simple but beneficial addition to our MTX educational program.

Author(s): Oakley, D., & Bogue, E.
Article Title: Quality of condom use as reported by female clients of a family planning clinic
Journal Title: *American Journal of Public Health*
Volume (Issue): 85(11)   **Year:** 1995 (November)   **Pages:** 1526–1530

Summary: This study analyzed the prevalence and determinants of the quality of condom use after a woman's first visit to a family planning clinic. This report presents data from 360 female family planning clients who reported using condoms as their primary method of contraception for at least 1 sexually active month during the study's follow-up period after their first clinic visit. Only 1% always engaged in all five use behaviors studied—using a condom for each sexual intercourse, putting the condom on before first entry, withdrawal after intercourse while there is still an erection, holding on to the condom's rim during withdrawal, and using foam. Multiple linear regression indicated that more effective condom use was reported by women who had not had an induced abortion, were not using condoms just because they were starting oral contraceptive pill regimens, had more knowledge about birth control in general, had received a nursing intervention, and had more communication with their partner.

Health Maintenance Organization (HMOs) (N = 2)

Author (s): Banks, N., Palmer, R., Berwick, D., & Plsek, P.
Article Title: Variability in clinical systems: Applying modern quality control methods to health care
Journal Title: *The Joint Commission Journal on Quality Improvement*
Volume (Issue): 21(8)   **Year:** 1995   **Pages:** 407–417

Summary: This study evaluated the concepts and tools of quality management for measuring system performance in ambulatory care. Clinical staff in nine centers of a group model health maintenance organization described the procedure for ordering and completing a complete blood count, mammogram, and surgical consultation. Variability was noted among the processes as intended and as actually performed, as well as inconsistencies reported within and among centers. Computerized patient records and departmental files were the only available sources of data for assessing completion and follow-up of tests and consultations. Although data were often difficult to obtain, the quality management techniques used were helpful in revealing process failures that appeared to be the result of design flaws built into the clinical systems.

Author(s): Hoare, K., Lacoste, J., Haro, K., & Conyers, C.
Article Title: Exploring indicators of telephone nursing quality
Journal Title: *Journal of Nursing Care Quality*
Volume (Issue): 14(1)   **Year:** 1999 (October)   **Pages:** 38–46

Summary: To explore whether documentation, use of clinical guidelines, and nurse competency are the best indicators of quality telephone nursing, this study examined the relationship between these commonly cited indicators and the characteristics of a telephone nursing call. This study, done at a large health maintenance organization (HMO) found: Accompanying symptoms played a major role in telephone nursing assessment; call length was related to documentation process and to number of visits to a health care facility after a call; nurses' interpersonal skills and ability to determine urgency of a call are related to the documentation process but not to outcomes of the call; time of a call is related to disposition; and disposition is related to number of visits after a call.

Nursing Center (N = 1)

Author(s): Adams, J., Kotarba, J.A., Wardell, D., Sherwood, G., Engebretson J., & Salmon, L.
Article Title: An ethnographic assessment of an academic nursing center
Journal Title: *Journal of the American Academy of Nurse Practitioners*
Volume (Issue): 8(8) **Year:** 1996 (August) **Pages:** 365–371

Summary: The purpose of this study was to provide a description and analysis of an academic nursing center. Through a series of observations and interviews, an interdisciplinary team investigated the history and organizational development of the center; the everyday delivery of services; staffing; and participants' assessment of the efficiency and quality of its services and recommendations for improving the services provided in the examined nursing center.

Community Health Nursing Quality Measurement Studies | 3

Overview

Although only 10 community health care studies were located, 7 focused on quality improvement projects for improving nursing care of specific clinical issues in this setting. Most of the studies focused on primary and secondary prevention strategies for child health, such as improving immunization rates, supporting breastfeeding, and treating childhood anemia. One study reported that commonly accepted outcome measures such as infant mortality, teen births, and immunization rates were used in most child health reports, but that process measures for quality improvement efforts were notably lacking (Halfon, Newacheck, Hughes, & Brindis, 1998). Another study evaluated the Maternal and Child Health Epidemiology Program (MCHEP) and concluded that overall, state health agencies appeared weakest in three components: the presence of adequately trained personnel, adequate management information systems to support MCH programs, and adequate understanding of the MCH planning cycle (Handler, Geller, & Kennelly, 1999). These two studies indicate that process and structural measures are not the usual focus of quality improvement efforts in this setting.

Only one study investigated process and structural variables in this setting. Walker, Baker, and Chiverton (1998) examined an activity-based costing methodology and the cost-effectiveness of primary care and mental health services provided by advanced practice nurses (APNs) in a school-based health center. A great deal of health care delivered by APNs in community-based settings includes primary and secondary prevention activities such as health promotion, screening, counseling, and anticipatory guidance. One area that needs further exploration is activity-based costing to identify actual costs of care (versus charges) in community health care settings where APNs deliver primary care.

In summary, quality improvement efforts in community health care have traditionally focused on outcome measures with little attention placed on process and structural variables such as staffing, information management, and cost.

These areas beg for further investigation and must be addressed in quality improvement projects.

The 10 community health nursing quality measurement studies in this chapter are organized as follows:

▌ Quality outcomes
▌ Program evaluation

Quality Outcomes (N = 7)

Author(s): Alexander, J., & Kroposki, M.
Article Title: Outcomes for community health nursing practice
Journal Title: *Journal of Nursing Administration*
Volume (Issue): 29(5)   Year: 1999 (May)   Pages: 49–56

Summary: The purpose of this study was to develop an easy, practical list of outcomes amenable to community health nursing interventions. A modified Delphi technique was used with three rounds of Delphi questionnaires generated from focus groups. Findings produced a list of 48 nursing outcomes in four domains: client's psychosocial components of care, client's physiologic components of care, nursing intervention/implementation components of care, and environmental/community safety components of care.

Author(s): Cleary, K.
Article Title: Using claims data to measure and improve the MMR immunization rate in an HMO
Journal Title: *The Joint Commission Journal on Quality Improvement*
Volume (Issue): 21(5)   Year: 1995   Pages: 211–217

Summary: This article describes how one HMO with more than 350,000 members set up a three-phase study to improve immunization compliance rates. Baseline MMR immunization compliance study yielded a rate 91.7%, which, as a first check of quality, is quite good in comparison to the nationally reported MMR compliance figures of 79.3% Analysis demonstrated that by seeking chart information, the overall MMR compliance rate was actually 96.7%. Reasons for noncompliance are described, as well as the process used and improvements made.

Author(s): Honnas, R., & Zlotnick, C.
Article Title: Quality improvement in action: Development of a tool
Journal Title: *Journal of Nursing Care Quality*
Volume (Issue): 9(4)   Year: 1995   Pages: 72–77

Summary: Based on findings of the Utilization/Peer Review Forum, a quality assurance system committee composed of public health professionals, there was question about whether public health nurses followed the standards of care when treating children with anemia. The article describes the process of identifying the problem and then developing and implementing an investigation to determine the magnitude of the problem. A sample of 703 child care records was audited; as a result of this process, conflicts in the established protocols of the county health department were identified, and an unexpectedly high prevalence of childhood anemia was discovered.

Author(s): Leff, E., Schriefer, J., Hagan, J., & DeMarco, P.
Article Title: Improving breastfeeding support: A community health improvement project
Journal Title: *The Joint Commission Journal on Quality Improvement*
Volume (Issue): 21(10)   **Year:** 1995   **Pages:** 521–529

Summary: In 1992, feedback from patients who had given birth suggested a need for more consistent, expert, and timely assistance with breastfeeding in the hospital and better continuity of care during the first few weeks at home. A team developed objectives, analyzed the problem and possible solutions, and made eight recommendations on how the hospital could do more to promote breastfeeding. Implementation by team members and hospital staff included policy development, staff education, acquisition of funding, a visiting professorship, development of a lactation consultant coordinator and team, and patient surveys to evaluate the program. A survey of 63 postpartum patients on their day of discharge indicated a high level of satisfaction with breastfeeding support in the hospital.

Author(s): Morriey-Ro, M., & Greiner, P.A.
Article Title: Hitting the mark in community health outreach: What counts?
Journal Title: *Journal for Healthcare Quality*
Volume (Issue): 22(1)   **Year:** 2000 (January/February)   **Pages:** 17–23

Summary: This article describes a nurse-managed community health outreach project designed to prevent cardiovascular disease in an inner city community. Early findings are presented as numbers of moderate- to high-risk cardiovascular patients identified and receiving follow-up intervention. Other indicators of project success being tracked include: The number of referrals, number of people triaged to emergency care, number of abnormal values that later improve to normal, client satisfaction at screenings and follow-up number of people found to have a health problem of which they were previously unaware, number of people who make behavioral changes due to screening and education, number of other health problems discovered as a result of nurse–patient interviews and referrals, and a decrease in morbidity and mortality rates for heart disease and stroke in the community.

Author(s): Van Acker, B., McIntosh, G., & Gudes, M.
Article Title: Continuous quality improvement techniques enhance HMO members' immunization rates
Journal Title: *Journal for Healthcare Quality*
Volume (Issue): 20(2)   **Year:** 1998   **Pages:** 36–41

Summary: To have a positive impact on the immunization rate of the 4000 newborn infants it covers each year, Blue Care Network of Southeast Michigan

(BCNSEM), a 240,000-member HMO based on an independent provider association model, convened a continuous quality improvement team. One of the results of this initiative was the development and implementation of an immunization registry, which is used as an internal tracking and reminder system for its members and providers. In recognition of its efforts, BCNSEM recently earned a Celebrating Innovation award from the American Association of Health Plans.

Author(s): Walker, P. H., Baker, J. J., & Chiverton, P.
Article Title: Costs of interdisciplinary practice in a school-based health center
Journal Title: *Outcomes Management for Nursing Practice*
Volume (Issue): 2(1) **Year:** 1998 (January–March) **Pages:** 37–44

Summary: In the context of market-driven health care reform, interest in cost and quality outcomes has increased. Quality, as defined by Donabedian (1988). Includes assessment of structure, process, and outcomes. However, the definition of quality in health care must be expanded to include the expectations and opinions of patients, their representatives, and society. The purpose of this article is to examine the outcome variable of costs in a specific nursing practice setting. Cost is frequently defined as the judicious use of resources consumed by structures and processes of care. This article presents activity-based costing methodology and results of a cost study of primary care and mental health services provided by APNs in a school-based health center. The application of the methods and outcomes of this pilot study has significant implications for the delivery of health care by APNs in a variety of settings, including community nursing centers, freestanding birthing centers, and rural and urban neighborhood centers. Because much of the health care delivered by APNs in these community-based settings includes health promotion, screening, counseling, and anticipatory guidance, it is important to explore methods such as activity-based costing to identify actual costs of care (versus charges) in emerging community-based practices where APNs deliver primary care.

Program Evaluation (N = 3)

Author(s): Halfon, N., Newacheck, P. W., Hughes, D., & Brindis, C.
Article Title: Community health monitoring: Taking the pulse of America's children
Journal Title: *Maternal & Child Health Journal*
Volume (Issue): 2(2) **Year:** 1998 (June) **Pages:** 95–109

Summary: To describe the development, content, enablers/barriers, and impact of child health reports in nine communities, a qualitative, prospective, multiyear, longitudinal evaluation used a multiple case study methodology. Three waves of structured in-person and telephone interviews of the project staff, community leaders, and key participants tracked the development of child health reports in all nine communities. A mailed survey of project directors was administered to assess accomplishments at the completion of the project. Content analysis of each community health report was conducted using different conceptual frameworks for health measurement and reporting. Although commonly accepted outcome measures were used in most reports (eg, infant mortality, teen births, immunization rates), process indicators, important for quality monitoring and community health improvement, were notably lacking. In each community, the reports were credited with providing a more comprehensive and integrated view of the health needs of children. Additional conceptual and technical work is needed to improve the ability of community health reports to capture key indicators of interest.

Author(s): Handler, A., Geller, S., & Kennelly, J.
Article Title: Effective MCH epidemiology in state health agencies: Lessons from an evaluation of the Maternal and Child Health Epidemiology Program (MCHEP)
Journal Title: *Maternal & Child Health Journal*
Volume (Issue): 3(4)   **Year:** 1999 (December)   **Pages:** 217–224

Summary: The Maternal and Child Health Epidemiology Program (MCHEP) was evaluated in 1996 and 1997. As part of this evaluation, an effort was undertaken to identify components of effective MCH epidemiology, examine their prevalence across participating states, and assess differences with respect to these components between MCHEP and non-MCHEP states. A case study evaluation was undertaken in which nine states (five MCHEP and four non-MCHEP) rated themselves on a benchmark questionnaire and participated in interviews conducted during site visits. Components on which the states appeared weakest overall were the presence of adequately trained personnel, the presence of adequate management information systems to support MCH programs, and whether the state health agency's epidemiologic unit understands the MCH planning cycle. There were seven components on which the two groups of states differed. These include whether the MCH director is empowered in the state health agency, whether the state health agency has identified internal epidemiologic capacity building as a priority, and whether analytic leadership is available for MCH epidemiologic activities.

Author(s): Lamb, G. S.
Article Title: Early lessons from a capitated community-based nursing model
Journal Title: *Nursing Administration Quarterly*
Volume (Issue): 19(3)   **Year:** 1995 (Spring)   **Pages:** 18–26

Summary: The community nursing organization (CNO) demonstration is a 3-year Medicare program to develop, manage, and evaluate a new capitated, nurse-managed system of community and ambulatory care. Since February 1994, four national sites have started CNOs. The CNO at Carondelet Health Care in Tucson, Arizona, shares early experiences in designing and implementing an exciting new community practice model.

Home Health Nursing Quality Measurement Studies 4

Overview

Since 1995, home health studies measuring quality have increased as compared to the findings of the previous review of nursing studies. Whereas only 19 home care studies were located previously (Rantz, 1995), this study identified 27 articles that focused on quality of nursing care in this setting. One third of the studies focused on quality outcome and quality improvement efforts; others investigated patient satisfaction, staff perceptions, and program evaluation or regulatory issues. Another third of the studies dealt with documentation, discharge planning, patient teaching, and case management in the home health setting. One article focused on an instrument designed to evaluate high-tech home care nursing processes. This is in sharp contrast to the previous study in which 78% of the studies (7 out of 9) dealt with instruments designed to measure the process and quality of nursing care in this setting (1995).

Total quality management (TQM), continuous quality improvement (CQI), and quality assurance (QA) principles are used in this setting to improve quality outcomes for home health care clients. One intervention study targeted medically ill older adults with symptoms of depression in order to reduce their rate of hospitalization (Flaherty et al., 1998). Although receiving mental health or geriatric nurse visits did not seem to lower hospitalization rates more than another, these interventions did approach statistical significance ($p = .052$) when compared with the control group. Another intervention study investigated medication compliance of community-dwelling elders (Fulmer et al., 1999). Telephone call reminders were found to be an important intervention in terms of enhancing medication compliance in this population.

With the rapid growth in the home health care industry, nurses are challenged by recent system changes to make effective use of their time during home visits. The use of cellular phones and computers in the field was proven useful as a productivity benchmark in the home care industry (Derrick, 1998). In addition, pay-per-visit payment was frequently mentioned in the surveys as a potential method to improve staff productivity and reduce costs for the agency (1998). The ever-changing regulatory environment of the home health industry has led to competitive agency behaviors, improved access to most services, changes in staffing patterns, and concerns for quality of care (Ellenbecker, 1995). Although the effect of recent system changes on nursing practice and patient care was not found to have an adverse affect on nurses and nursing care, some troubling trends were suggested (Ellenbecker & Warren, 1998).

As found in the previous review of nursing quality studies (Rantz, 1995), discharge planning and patient satisfaction continue to be of major concern in this setting. Dimensions of care most closely associated with overall perceptions of quality were identified via discriminant analysis for the purpose of developing quality indices for use in CQI initiatives (Kansky & Brannon, 1996).

In summary, rapid growth, change in reimbursement regulations, the use of technology, and concerns regarding improvement in quality outcomes are the focus of important research in this field. Patient and staff satisfaction remain closely linked to discharge arrangements, easy access, affordable costs, flexible scheduling, and quality nursing care and are likely to be the focus of on-going research.

The 27 home health nursing quality measurement studies in this chapter are organized as follows:

- Quality outcomes/quality improvement
- Patient satisfaction/staff perceptions
- Program evaluation/regulatory
- Documentation/OASIS
- Discharge planning/patient teaching
- Case management/critical paths
- Instruments

Quality Outcomes/Quality Improvement (N = 8)

Author(s): Adams, C. E., Kramer, S., & Wilson, M.
Article Title: Home health quality outcomes: Fee-for-service versus health maintenance organization enrollees
Journal Title: *Journal of Nursing Administration*
Volume (Issue): 25(11) **Year:** 1995 **Pages:** 39–45

Summary: Quality outcomes were compared between home health patients enrolled in the traditional Medicare fee-for-service (FFS) program versus a health maintenance organization (HMO) with a Medicare cost contract with the federal government. The quality outcome scores were similar between the two patient groups. However, the other home health research showed superior quality outcomes for patients enrolled in the traditional Medicare FFS program versus an HMO with a risk contract with the federal government. Before signing contracts with HMOs, home health administrators will want to identify the type of Medicare contract the HMO has with the federal government.

Author(s): Ellenbecker, C. H.

Article Title: Profit and non-profit home health care agency outcomes: A study of one state's experience

Journal Title: *Home Health Care Services Quarterly*

Volume (Issue): 15(3)   **Year:** 1995   **Pages:** 47–60

Summary: The purpose of this study was to describe differences in behaviors and industry outcomes generated by nonprofit and for-profit organizations in Massachusetts. Data for the study were from the Massachusetts State Department of Public Health's Annual Reports of Home Health Agencies. Results suggest that although for-profit and nonprofit agencies behave similarly in many areas, there are areas of difference, with significant differences found in the amount of service delivered and the rates charged.

Author(s): Flaherty, J. H., McBride, M., Marzouk, S., Miller, D. K., Chien, N., Hanchett, M., Leander, S., Kaiser, F. E., & Morley, J. E.

Article Title: Decreasing hospitalization rates for older home care patients with symptoms of depression

Journal Title: *Journal of the American Geriatrics Society*

Volume (Issue): 46(1)   **Year:** 1998 (January)   **Pages:** 31–38

Summary: A case-control study was conducted to target medically ill older home care patients with symptoms of depression to reduce their rate of hospitalization. Home care patients 65 years of age and older with symptoms of depression who were participants of a TQM intervention ($n = 81$) were compared with an historical control of home care patients 65 years of age and older with symptoms of depression ($n = 69$). The TQM intervention patients had a higher mean age than the historical control patients but were not different in percent female, percent white race, percent with a caregiver in the home, functional status, and in 15 of 16 diagnostic categories. Overall, the TQM intervention group had a hospitalization rate of 23.5% (19/81) compared with a rate of 40.6% (28/69) for the historical control group ($p = .024$). One type of intervention did not seem to lower hospitalization rates more than another although having received the MH or GN visits approached significance (12/50, 24%; $p = .052$) when compared with the control group. Using TQM principles and the development of an intervention such as the one described here can decrease hospitalization rates for medically ill older home care patients with symptoms of depression.

Author(s): Fulmer, T. T., Feldman, P. H., Kim, T. S., Carty, B., Beers, M., Molina, M., & Putnam, M.

Article Title: An intervention study to enhance medication compliance in community-dwelling elderly individuals

Journal Title: *Journal of Gerontological Nursing*

Volume (Issue): 25(8)   **Year:** 1999 (August)   **Pages:** 6–14

Summary: Medication compliance for community-dwelling elderly individuals is a complex process. Currently, there are a variety of strategies that are categorized as enabling, consequence, and stimulant. Telephone call reminders are an important intervention in terms of enhancing medication compliance in community-dwelling elderly individuals. Technological advances show promise for even stronger intervention in the future.

Author(s): Kane, R. A., Frytak, J., & Eustis, N. N.
Article Title: Agency approaches to common quality problems in home care: A scenario study
Journal Title: *Home Health Care Services Quarterly*
Volume (Issue): 16(1/2)   **Year:** 1997   **Pages:** 21–40

Summary: In a study of best practices in home care QA, a sample of 128 respondents from exemplary home care agencies were presented with seven brief scenarios depicting common problems in home care quality. Agency respondents were asked to describe their likelihood of identifying the problem in each scenario, how they would identify the problem, and how they would correct it. We found that agencies expressed considerable confidence they would identify the problems, but were unlikely to view their QA efforts as contributing to detecting the problems. Identification was more often perceived to come from ordinary care, with considerable burden placed on paraprofessional staff or clients to bring the problem to the attention of the agency. Medically oriented agencies were significantly more likely than socially oriented agencies to rely on formal QA to identify deteriorating patient conditions and depression. Across all agencies, a relationship existed between the type of problem in the scenario and the most frequent responses about detection and correction modes. Once the problem was identified, agencies presented an appropriate and fairly wide range of corrective strategies. The implications for making QA more organically related to clinical care are discussed.

Author(s): Kendra, M. A., & Weiker, A.
Article Title: Chart audit using the American Nurses Association standards of practice
Journal Title: *Home Healthcare Nurse*
Volume (Issue): 14(7)   **Year:** 1996 (July)   **Pages:** 551–556

Summary: This article describes a study using chart audits as a strategy for CQI within a home health agency's quality improvement program. Findings are discussed using the American Nurses Association Standards of Home Health Nursing Practice as a framework.

Author(s): Lee, T. T., & Mills, M. E.
Article Title: Analysis of patient profile in predicting home care resource utilization and outcomes
Journal Title: *Journal of Nursing Administration*
Volume (Issue): 30(2)   **Year:** 2000 (February)   **Pages:** 67–75

Summary: This study identified patient profile variables that can explain variation in resource utilization and outcomes for home health care. A retrospective descriptive study design was used in which patient records ($n = 244$) data were obtained from a home health care agency in Washington D.C. A series of stepwise and discriminant analyses indicates that data related to nursing diagnoses and nursing interventions can provide valuable in predicting resource use. Prognosis made by nursing judgment was also found to be sensitive in predicting patient outcomes.

Author(s): Phillips, L. R., Morrison, E., Steffl, B., Chae, Y. M., Cromwell, S. L., & Russell, C. K.
Article Title: Effects of the situational context and interactional process on the quality of family caregiving
Journal Title: *Research in Nursing & Health*
Volume (Issue): 18(3) **Year:** 1995 **Pages:** 205–216

Summary: To test the family caregiving dynamics model (FCDM), designed to explain variation in quality of elder care (QEC) for those receiving care at home from family caregivers. Data were collected using interviews, observations, and self-reports. Two hundred nine elder–caregiver dyads comprised the sample. These findings support the assumption that caregiving burden contributes to poor QEC and in the way predicted. It also mediates the relationship between QEC and factors in the situational context and interactional process. The explanatory power of burden, however, decreased as situational and interactional variables were added to the model. This may indicate that burden is a proxy for other factors affecting the caregiving situation. Second, the findings suggest that the situational context is not as strong a predictor of QEC as conventional wisdom suggests. Of the situational variables, only activities of daily living (ADL) had a direct effect on QEC. Third, these findings suggest the interactional process strongly affects QEC.

Patient Satisfaction/Staff Perceptions (N = 6)

Author(s): Ellenbecker, C. H., & Warren, K.
Article Title: Nursing practice and patient care in a changing home healthcare environment
Journal Title: *Home Healthcare Nurse*
Volume (Issue): 16(8) **Year:** 1998 (August) **Pages:** 531–539

Summary: The home health care industry is in a period of rapid growth and change driven by events occurring in the larger health care system. This descriptive, qualitative study explored the effect of recent system changes on home health care nurses and their practice. Nurses in six focus groups contributed data on their perceptions of these effects. Study results suggest that nurses and nursing care have not been adversely affected by recent system changes. However, results also suggest some troubling trends.

Author(s): Foley, M. E., Fahs, M. C., Eisenhandler, J., & Hyer, K.
Article Title: Satisfaction with home healthcare services for clients with HIV: Preliminary findings
Journal Title: *Journal of the Association of Nurses in AIDS Care*
Volume (Issue): 6(5) **Year:** 1995 **Pages:** 20–25

Summary: The Visiting Nurse Service of New York and Empire Blue Cross and Blue Shield implemented the "At Home Options Program" (AHOP) in 1990, an enhanced package of home care and other non-inpatient services for HIV-positive clients. AHOP aims to reduce total treatment costs and hospital days. Clients ($N = 52$) completed mailed satisfaction surveys. Overall, clients were very satisfied with AHOP services. Clients expressed concerns, however, about the uneven quality of substitute paraprofessionals, and said they needed easier access to a knowledgeable health care professional. Operational concerns included inadequate information dissemination and administrative oversights. Findings will inform subsequent program activities.

Author(s): Kansky, K. H., & Brannon, D.
Article Title: Discriminant analysis: A technique for adding value to patient satisfaction surveys
Journal Title: *Hospital & Health Services Administration*
Volume (Issue): 41(4) **Year:** 1996 (Winter) **Pages:** 503–513

Summary: This paper describes a methodology that identifies dimensions of care most closely associated with overall perceptions of quality. A patient satisfaction survey was mailed to 2055 discharged patients of 13 home health agencies. Patients were asked to evaluate service dimensions of home health relating to scheduling, nursing care, home health aide services, and discharge arrangements. Overall satisfaction with quality of services was used as the dependent variable in two discriminant analysis equations. Eleven dimensions discriminated between "excellent" and "good" quality, and seven dimensions discriminated between "satisfactory" and "unsatisfactory" quality. Using discriminant analysis, items most closely associated with quality indices can be identified and used in CQI initiatives.

Author(s): Kendra, M. A., Weiker, A., Simon, S., Grant, A., & Shullick, D.
Article Title: Safety concerns affecting delivery of home health care
Journal Title: *Public Health Nursing*
Volume (Issue): 13(2) **Year:** 1996 (April) **Pages:** 83–89

Summary: The purpose of this pilot study was to ascertain factors related to perception of risk by home health care administrators and staff and determine whether quality of care is affected when home-visit situations present risk. A convenience sample of 36 home health care administrators and 62 staff was surveyed about risks and measures provided by the home health care agency to minimize risk. Factors associated with risk are geographic location, high incidence of crime, inappropriate patient or caregiver behavior, infectious diseases, and evening assignments. Strategies used to minimize risk include safety programs, preplanning of visits, personal protective equipment, escorts, and buddy systems. Perceived ability to refuse high-risk assignments, however, is questionable; 66% of the staff stated that they leave a situation "as soon as possible." These findings will be used to strengthen in-service programs and to provide a basis for future studies

Author(s): Piercy, K. W., & Woolley, D. N.
Article Title: Negotiating worker–client relationships: A necessary step to providing quality home health care
Journal Title: *Home Health Care Services Quarterly*
Volume (Issue): 18(1)   **Year:** 1999   **Pages:** 1–24

Summary: A qualitative study was conducted to investigate definitions of quality home health care and how good quality care was achieved from consumer and provider perspectives. Using semi-structured interviews, members of 16 families and their home health aides described the skills required for good quality care. Although able performance of essential tasks was considered part of quality care, relational skills of home health aides were crucial to good quality care. Relationships were negotiated between worker and client that were characterized as close and preserving of client autonomy. When such relationships were achieved, workers were frequently described as insiders in client families. High performing aides also undergo a process of intrapersonal negotiation to give meaning to their work. Implications for recruitment and training of home health aides and for measuring quality care in home health are discussed.

Author(s): Riccio, P. A.
Article Title: Quality evaluation of home nursing care: Perceptions of patients, physicians, and nurses
Journal Title: *Nursing Administration Quarterly*
Volume (Issue): 24(3)   **Year:** 2000 (Spring)   **Pages:** 43–52

Summary: Perceptions of patients ($n = 135$), physicians ($n = 99$), and nurses ($n = 20$) regarding home nursing care were studied using a descriptive survey conducted over a 6-month period in a large, voluntary, nonprofit home health agency. An original instrument, based on the American Nurses Association standards of home nursing care within a nursing process framework, was developed for this study. Factor analyses (varimax rotation) yielded four subscales: technical, professional, communication/psychosocial, and teaching aspects of nursing care. Overall, patients and physicians rated their satisfaction with nursing care identically (20% were satisfied, 71% were undecided, 9% were dissatisfied); whereas 70% of the nurses were satisfied, 20% were undecided, and 10% were dissatisfied with their nursing care. Both physicians and patients were most satisfied with professional aspects of nursing care; nurses were most satisfied with teaching aspects. Patients and physicians were most dissatisfied with teaching; nurses were equally dissatisfied with technical skills and communication/psychosocial aspects of nursing care.

Program Evaluation/Regulatory (N = 4)

Author(s): Derrick, A. M.
Article Title: Research corner. Benchmarking productivity in home health care
Journal Title: *Home Health Care Management & Practice*
Volume (Issue): 10(3)   **Year:** 1998 (April)   **Pages:** 71–77

Summary: This descriptive study was developed to identify what productivity benchmarks are being used in the home care industry today. Staff productivity was measured in terms of the number of visits performed per discipline in an 8-hour workday. Information was also gathered on what activities were taking place in the home care agencies to improve staff productivity. A survey was developed by the benchmarking team to collect qualitative and quantitative data. The results show the majority of home care agencies who responded pay staff on an hourly basis. Pay/visit payment was frequently mentioned in the surveys as a potential method to improve staff productivity and reduce costs for the agency. Eighty percent reported using cellular phones and 20% reported using computers in the field. No significant relationship between mileage and staff productivity was found.

Author(s): Ellenbecker, C. H.
Article Title: Home health care industry growth and change: A study of one state's experience
Journal Title: *Home Health Care Services Quarterly*
Volume (Issue): 15(3)   **Year:** 1995   **Pages:** 61–81

Summary: This is a descriptive study of one state's experience with a changing regulatory environment over a 10-year period of time. Data from the Massachusetts Department of Public Health's Annual Reports for Home Health Agencies were used to describe industry growth and change, and the effect these had on the accessibility, quality, and efficiency of service delivery from 1980 to 1990. Results suggest dramatic changes in the industry, with strong evidence of agencies' competitive behaviors, improved patient access to most services, changes in staffing patterns, and concerns for quality of care.

Author(s): Jette, A. M., Smith, K. W., & McDermott, S. M.
Article Title: Quality of Medicare-reimbursed home health care
Journal Title: *Gerontologist*
Volume (Issue): 36(4)   **Year:** 1996   **Pages:** 492–501

Summary: The prevalence of quality of care deficiencies in 4324 Medicare-reimbursed episodes of care provided by 47 home health agencies was investigated. The quality of care protocol consisted of a process-oriented, systematic record review by a trained nurse reviewer. Results suggest that an estimated 14.4% of home health care episodes had quality deficiencies with the potential for or actual adverse effects on the patient. Multivariate analyses revealed that the complexity of patients' needs increased the likelihood and severity of the quality problems. Agency ownership was not related to risk of a quality problem, but regional variation in agency effects was observed. Specific problem areas were identified that suggested several ways that home health care could be improved.

Author(s): Schlenker, R. E., Hittle, D. F., & Arnold, A. G.
Article Title: Home health agency quality: Medicare certification findings compared to patient outcomes

Journal Title: *Home Health Care Services Quarterly*
Volume (Issue): 15(4) **Year:** 1995 **Pages:** 97–115

Summary: As part of an evaluation of the Medicare certification program for home health agencies (HHAs), the extent to which certification findings were related to patient outcomes was examined. In a previous study, longitudinal patient data for a national sample of 42 HHAs were collected and precise patient outcome measures were developed. In this study, the outcome measures were compared to certification findings for the same HHAs and time period (1991 to 1993). There was relatively little association between the two sets of measures. The findings indicate that the Medicare HHA survey process does not yet successfully incorporate patient outcomes.

Documentation/OASIS (N = 4)

Author(s): Adams, C. E., Wilson, M., Haney, M., & Short, R.
Article Title: Using the outcome-based quality improvement model and OASIS to improve HMO patients' outcomes
Journal Title: *Home Healthcare Nurse*
Volume (Issue): 16(6) **Year:** 1998 (June) **Pages:** 395–401

Summary: The study purpose was to determine if use of the Outcome-Based Quality Improvement (OBQI) model, including a subset of the Outcome Assessment and Information Set (OASIS), enhanced outcomes for HMO patients referred for care to six contracted HHAs. After four quarters of data-driven QI activities, the improvement scores of the patients were not changed significantly from the baseline period. Stabilization scores increased significantly for two of the five outcome measures. Use of OASIS and the OBQI model for HMO patients referred to multiple HHAs requires that contracted HHAs share outcome results and quality improvement conclusions.

Author(s): Adams, C. E., & Wilson, M.
Article Title: Enhanced quality through outcome-focused standardized care plans
Journal Title: *Journal of Nursing Administration*
Volume (Issue): 25(9) **Year:** 1995 **Pages:** 27–34

Summary: Methods to improve the quality of care are a national issue for home health care agencies. In comparison with the traditional process-focused care plans, outcome-focused care plans (OCPs) resulted in significantly better quality indicator scores for clients cared for by agency staff members. Although OCPs are a valuable tool for enhancing quality, tools are only as good as the individuals who use them. Before deciding to change to an OCP format, administrators must assess all resources needed to effect the change.

Author(s): Adams, C. E., DeFrates, D. S., & Wilson, M.
Article Title: Data-driven quality improvement for HMO patients
Journal Title: *Journal of Nursing Administration*
Volume (Issue): 28(10) **Year:** 1998 (October) **Pages:** 20–25

Summary: The authors determined whether a home health agency could use OASIS items and the OBQI model to enhance outcomes for HMO patients. After an initial baseline period and four quarters of quality improvement activities, improvement and stabilization scores showed few significant changes. When the results were reviewed, investigators considered both the HMO authorization patterns and challenges encountered in using the OASIS–OBQI paradigm.

Author(s): Borchers, E. L.
Article Title: Improving nursing documentation for private-duty home health care
Journal Title: *Journal of Nursing Care Quality*
Volume (Issue): 13(5)   **Year:** 1999 (June)   **Pages:** 24–43, 91–92

Summary: Private duty home health care agencies have struggled to ensure compliance with accurate and complete nursing documentation. In this descriptive study, the author reports on an improvement and innovation project in a private duty, home health care agency aimed at improving nursing documentation, as measured in chart review audits. Initial strategies were directed toward revising the documentation system, with implementation of a flow record, and conducting group nurse education. These efforts had a minimal effect on improving documentation compliance. A major, multifocus strategy was then implemented. The educational component stressed pre- and posttest. The chart audit tool was revised to track individual nurse behaviors. Nurses were mentored when documentation did not meet standards. Last, the nurse job description and corresponding performance appraisal document were revised to clarify nurse responsibility and strengthen nurse accountability; progressive discipline was initiated when warranted. Significant and sustained improvement was subsequently realized.

Discharge Planning/Patient Teaching (N = 2)

Author(s): Arford, P. H., Michel, Y., McCue, P. S., & Hiott, B.
Article Title: Quality and cost outcomes of transitional care
Journal Title: *Nursing Economics*
Volume (Issue): 14(5)   **Year:** 1996 (September–October)   **Pages:** 266–275

Summary: Longitudinal analysis of the outcomes of a transitional care program documented success in discharging patients to home with remarkable compliance with discharge plans and sustained improvement in mental status and functional independence. Inpatient costs were significantly reduced.

Author(s): Hanstine, S., & Fanning, V.
Article Title: Teaching patients to manage diabetes safely in the home
Journal Title: *Home Health Care Management & Practice*
Volume (Issue): 12(4)   **Year:** 2000 (June)   **Pages:** 40–48

Summary: Using an interdisciplinary process improvement team approach, the average patient's diabetic knowledge improved 27% during the episode of care.

This improvement was accomplished by creating a pre-/posttest that could also be used as a teaching tool.

Case Management/Critical Paths (N = 2)

Author(s): Currie, G. A., Brofman, L., & Saharia, A. N.
Article Title: American Subacute Care Association. Outcomes-based home health care improves results for patients with CHF
Journal Title: *Home Care Provider*
Volume (Issue): 2(3)   **Year:** 1997 (June)   **Pages:** 143–147

Summary: This article describes the results of a case study to assess the effectiveness of the InterPath care management system. The study focused on home care patients with congestive heart failure (CHF) and demonstrated the effectiveness of using an integrated process of critical pathways, outcome measures, and concurrent outcomes monitoring to improve results and lower care costs.

Author(s): Malnory, M.
Article Title: Mother–infant home care drives quality in a managed care environment
Journal Title: *Journal of Nursing Care Quality*
Volume (Issue): 11(4)   **Year:** 1997 (April)   **Pages:** 9–26

Summary: Advocates of inpatient managed care employing clinical pathways are confident that this patient management strategy reduces cost and promotes equivalent patient outcomes. Other health care professionals are concerned that cost reductions place patients at higher risk for adverse health events. Research is needed to demonstrate the true impact of cost-containment strategies on clinical outcomes. The article describes a study in progress comparing patients conventionally managed by their physicians with similar patients whose overall management involved a nurse case manager. This study explores the issue of resource costs that can be linked to clinical and financial outcome measures.

Instruments (N = 1)

Author(s): Davis, J. H.
Article Title: Total parenteral nutrition (TPN) at home: Prototype high-tech home care nursing
Journal Title: *Gastroenterology Nursing*
Volume (Issue): 19(6)   **Year:** 1996 (November–December)   **Pages:** 207–209

Summary: This study explored the cognitive, technical, and interpersonal components included in total parenteral nutrition (TPN) home care nursing. The purpose of this study was to evaluate psychometrically the Schmele Instrument to Measure the Process of Nursing Practice in Home Health (SIMP-H) so that it may be used to examine high-tech home care nursing processes. Home visits must be observed to identify the specific cognitive, technical, and interpersonal components included in high-tech home care nursing that are important for patient care outcomes. This study captured high-tech home care nursing process on videotape, which provided a medium for evaluating interobserver reliability fore the SIMP-H. Results revealed an interobserver reliability coefficient of .72.

Hospital-Based Nursing Quality Measurement Studies 5

Overview

Consistent with the 1995 review, the largest and most diverse group of quality measurement studies involved the hospital-based setting. The trend toward multidisciplinary approaches to quality has continued and been expanded (Alexander & Stone, 2000; Brickman, Axelrod, Roberson, & Flanagan, 1998). Reports of the development, implementation, and evaluation of clinical pathways for a variety of patient groups were numerous, with many of these projects involving multidisciplinary teams (Aspling & Lagoe, 1995; Waters et al., 1999). Collaboration between researchers and clinicians is also evident (Redmond, Riggleman, Sorrell, & Zerull, 1999). Although nurse-authors have continued to measure outcomes at the individual and unit-based level, a significant number of studies during this period also examined quality in broader contexts, across and among organizations. Quality improvement and evaluation methodologies for use across organizations have been described, such as Structured Implicit Review (SIR) (Pearson et al., 2000), the FADE method (Barton, Danek, Johns, & Coons, 1998), and the Uniform Data System for Medical Rehabilitation (UDS MR) in the rehabilitation hospital setting (Harmon, Sheehy, & Davis, 1998). In addition, a variety of timely health care system issues have been studied by nurse-authors and multidisciplinary groups. These issues include organizational restructuring and redesign, changing care delivery models, and the impact of the work environment on quality.

A wide range of quality outcome indicators were included in this body of literature. Traditional quality outcome indicators, including hospital readmission, length of stay, and mortality, were used extensively. Although limitations to outcome measures such as mortality have been identified (Franklin & Legault, 1999), these outcomes continue to be measured, in part due to the wide availability of these data within and across acute care settings. A variety of adverse occurrences, including medication error rates, patient falls, pressure ulcers, infections, and patient complaints, were also used as quality outcome measures in many of the studies reviewed, and relationships among such adverse occurrences have been examined (Blegen & Vaughn, 1998). Although selected outcome measures for each study were appropriate and clearly operationalized by authors, inconsistent reporting of adverse occurrences (Elnitsky, Nichols, & Palmer, 1997) and other measurement issues across diverse hospital-based settings (Wakefield et al., 1996) have made the collection of aggregate data problematic.

To facilitate the collection of consistent aggregate data and demonstrate links between nursing care and patient outcomes, in 1994 the ANA launched the Nursing Report Card Project. From the first phase of this project, 10 nursing-sensitive quality indicators (QIs) for the acute care setting were identified. The National Database of Nursing Quality Indicators (NDNQI), which remains under development, serves as a repository for facility data related to these 10 QIs. The QIs address the following: staff skill mix and staffing levels; maintenance of skin integrity (pressure ulcers); patient injury rate (falls); nosocomial infection rate; nursing staff satisfaction; and patient satisfaction with pain management, educational information, overall care, and nursing care.

The ANA Report Card for Nursing has the potential to provide consistent aggregate data and a nursing focus to the study of quality. It has also been suggested that more nurse-sensitive quality outcomes be measured using data elements from the Nursing Minimum Data Set (NMDS) (Rantz, 1995). The potential of these measures, however, has yet to be realized. Although further development of the NOC has occurred (Maas, Johnson, Moorhead, 1996), only one small exploratory hospital-based study was identified with the stated purpose of studying elements of the NMDS (Blewitt & Jones, 1996). Four studies were found with the intent of testing ANA quality indicators in acute care. Two of these projects involved statewide initiatives, in Texas and Virginia (Grobe et al., 1998; Sorrell & Redmond, 1997).

Although not explicitly identified, all of the ANA QIs were evident in the literature reviewed but received different amounts of attention. As in other settings, patient and caregiver satisfaction with overall care or with nursing care was an important indicator. An outcome variable in a number of additional studies related to care processes and specific patient populations. Pain management and patient satisfaction with pain management were also studied in some depth. However, only one of the reviewed studies dealt with patient education (Patyk, Gaynor & Verdin, 2000). Other ANA QIs such as skin integrity and patient falls also received minimal attention.

A number of variables related to organizational structure are also reflective of the ANA staff QIs. Staffing was addressed as it related to patient outcomes (Blegen & Vaughn, 1998; Lichtig, Knauf, & Milholland, 1999; Sochalski, Estabrooks, & Humphrey, 1999), staffing patterns (Luther & Walsh, 1999; Minnick & Pabst, 1998), and the use of float and agency staff (Strzalka & Havens, 1996). Nursing staff satisfaction has received minimal attention and the collection of staffing data has been very problematic (Grobe et al., 1998). A few studies reviewed staff perceptions and attitudes, and others compared and contrasted perceptions of staff and patients. Only one study included in this review examined the relationship between nurse job satisfaction and patient satisfaction with nursing care (Kangas, Kee, & McKee-Waddle, 1999). Another study examined the role of the nurse-practitioner in acute care (Knaus et al., 1997).

The 175 hospital-based nursing quality measurement studies in this chapter are organized as follows:

- Quality outcome measures
- Methods of quality measurement
- Case management/clinical pathways
- Patient safety
- Pain and pain management
- Care delivery models
- Staff and staffing
- Organizational restructure/redesign
- Infection control
- Specific clinical issues related to patient populations
- Clinical issues related to care processes
- Work environment
- Perceptions of quality
- Patient/caregiver satisfaction
- Technology use
- Patient education

Quality Outcome Measures (N = 16)

Author(s): Cullen, D., Bates, D., Small, S., Cooper, J., Nemeskai, A., & Leape, L.
Article Title: The incident reporting system does not detect adverse drug events: A problem for quality improvement
Journal Title: *The Joint Commission Journal on Quality Improvement*
Volume (Issue): 21(10)   **Year:** 1995   **Pages:** 541–552

Summary: The objectives of this study were to determine the frequency with which adverse drug events result in an incident report in hospitalized patients, and to determine if there were differences between quality assurance administrators, nurse leaders in quality assurance, and staff nurses as to whether an incident report should or would be filed for each adverse drug event. All patients admitted to five patient care units in one academic tertiary care hospital were studied between February and July of 1993. Of 54 adverse drug events identified by the study, only three patients (6%) had a corresponding incident report submitted to the hospital's quality assurance program or called into the pharmacy hotline. Voluntary reporting identified only a small fraction of adverse drug events. Using incident reports for quality assurance/quality improvement will lead to significant bias when assessing quality of care.

Author(s): Czarnecki, M. T.
Article Title: Benchmarking: A data-oriented look at improving health care performance
Journal Title: *Journal of Nursing Care Quality*
Volume (Issue): 10(3)   **Year:** 1996 (April)   **Pages:** 1–6

Summary: Benchmarking uses measures of comparative performance to develop an understanding of what is possible and how others have achieved higher levels of performance. Companies measure each other's performance, identify the best performer out of a group, and then seek to identify and understand the practices that can improve both clinical and administrative operations. When a powerful consortium of Cincinnati businesses began addressing ways to lower the cost of employee health care in a project known as the Iameter study, the University of Cincinnati Hospital joined the effort to identify and improve major cost factors. One aspect highlighted by this review is the length of stay in the neonatal intensive care unit (NICU). The results of the study were incorporated into an NICU early discharge program, which has had a number of positive effects in both patient care quality and cost containment.

Author(s): Dearmin, Brenner, J., & Migliori, R.
Article Title: Reporting on QI efforts for internal and external customers
Journal Title: *The Joint Commission Journal on Quality Improvement*
Volume (Issue): 21(6)   **Year:** 1995   **Pages:** 277–288

Summary: Data on sentinel events and outcomes analysis of a variety of clinical and administrative functions have assisted in identifying opportunities for improvement. For example, this hospital monitors the 5-year survival rate for patients with myocardial infarction (MI). With the adoption of treatment with streptokinase, data indicated frequent hypotension. Increase of infusion from 30 to 60 minutes led to a decrease in hypotension. By increasing the visibility of quality indicators (QIs) within the hospital, the internal quality reports have helped generate further QI activity, and the external report augmented further positive publicity among the local health care press. The reports are proven effective tools for communicating the hospital's ability to sustain and improve the quality of its services over time.

Author(s): Elnitsky, C., Nichols, B., & Palmer, K.
Article Title: Are hospital incidents being reported?
Journal Title: *Journal of Nursing Administration*
Volume (Issue): 27(11)   **Year:** 1997 November   **Pages:** 40–46

Summary: Risk management and quality improvement measures assume that staff recognize and report individual hospital incidents. A survey of nurses working in acute care hospitals in 15 localities across a southeastern state was conducted to explore nurses' hospital incident reporting behaviors and supervisors' beliefs about and use of incident reports. Nurse-managers may have reason to be concerned about this quality measure: the number of incidents documented may represent only a portion of all incidents.

Author(s): Franklin, P.D., & Legault, J.P.
Article Title: Using data to evaluate hospital inpatient mortality
Journal Title: *Journal of Nursing Care Quality*
Volume (Issue): Special issue no. 1   **Year:** 1999 (November)   **Pages:** 55–66

Summary: This article evaluates the use of hospital inpatient mortality as an indicator of health care outcomes and describes the development of related data. It demonstrates both the strengths and limitations of mortality as a measure of outcomes. It provides guidance concerning the development of raw and severity adjusted mortality data. It also provides information concerning data related to unexpected mortality and complications.

Author(s): Grobe, S. J., Becker, H., Calvin, A., Biering, P., Jordan, C., & Tabone, S.
Article Title: Clinical data for use in assessing quality: Lessons learned from the Texas Nurses' Association Report Card Project
Journal Title: *Seminars for Nurse Managers*
Volume (Issue): 6(3)   **Year:** 1998 (September)   **Pages:** 126–138

Summary: The purpose of this report is to describe the Texas Nurses' Association Report Card Project. As part of the American Nurses Association's (ANA) Safety and Quality Initiative, the project was designed as a feasibility study to determine whether clinically based quality indicator data could be collected in standard ways across acute care agencies in Texas. Clinicians from 12 agencies, under leadership of the professional association (Texas Nurses' Association), participated in this initial effort to reach consensus on clinical indicator definitions and on how to collect clinical data for each indicator. Data were collected for falls and injuries, bacteremias, pressure ulcers, skill mix, nursing hours per patient day, patient satisfaction (with nursing, hospital stay, education, and pain management), and nurse satisfaction. The process used is described, as well as the findings and the lessons learned. The importance of standard definitions and precise and standard primary sources for the data are emphasized for the phase II report card efforts to follow.

Author(s): Lagoe, R. J., Noetscher, C. M., & Murphy, M. E.
Article Title: Combined benchmarking of hospital outcomes and utilization
Journal Title: *Nursing Economics*
Volume (Issue): 18(2)   **Year:** March–April 2000   **Pages:** 63–70

Summary: A number of hospitals in two distinctly different geographic health care environments (California and New York) were studied to determine the differences in outcomes and utilization for three of the most common high-cost diagnostic-related groups (DRGs). Unscheduled hospital readmissions (within 30 days of initial discharge) were used as outcome indicators. Benchmark targets were established for patients with a diagnosis of congestive heart failure (CHF), acute MI treated medically, or chronic obstructive pulmonary disease (COPD) using scattergrams that showed each hospital's mean acute length of stay (LOS) on the x axis and the readmission rates on the y axis. "Benchmarks were identified as those points with the lowest values for both indicators, as demonstrated by points that were closest to the intersection of the two axes."

Author(s): Lagoe, R. J., Noetscher, C. M., Hohner, V. K., & Schmidt, G. M.
Article Title: Analyzing hospital readmissions using statewide discharge databases
Journal Title: *Journal of Nursing Care Quality*
Volume (Issue): 13(6)   **Year:** August 1999   **Pages:** 57–67

Summary: Hospital readmissions are an important indicator of the outcomes of care as well as a source of unnecessary health care expenditures. This study focused on development of a uniform algorithm for identification of hospital readmission data. It involved development of a uniform definition of readmissions that could be applied to multiple statewide computer databases. Through this approach, comparable readmission data were generated for use in benchmarking and quality improvement activities.

Author(s): Lagoe, R. J., Noetscher, C. M., & Murphy, M. E.
Article Title: Hospital readmissions at the community level: Implications for case management
Journal Title: *Journal of Nursing Care Quality*
Volume (Issue): 14(4)   **Year:** July 2000   **Pages:** 1–15

Summary: This study describes the development of information concerning the distribution of hospital readmissions by diagnosis in seven different U.S. metropolitan areas. The data demonstrated that circulatory disorders were associated with the largest number of community-wide readmissions in all of the communities. It also showed that circulatory, respiratory, and digestive disorders accounted for a majority of readmissions in all of the areas. This information suggested that case management efforts to reduce readmissions can focus on a limited range of clinical diagnoses. This approach should enable the process to function effectively within resource constraints.

Author(s): Mark, B. A., & Burleson, D. L.
Article Title: Measurement of patient outcomes: Data availability and consistency across hospitals
Journal Title: *Journal of Nursing Administration*
Volume (Issue): 25(4)   **Year:** 1995   **Pages:** 52–59

Summary: In a random sample of 20 hospitals, the availability and consistency of five patient outcome indicators were examined, including medication administration errors, patient falls, occurrence of new decubitus ulcers, nosocomial infections, and unplanned readmission to the hospital. The results indicate that information about only two outcome indicators—medication errors and patient falls—were collected consistently by the sampled hospitals. The findings are discussed in the context of implications for the study of patient outcomes research.

Author(s): McKay, M. D., Rowe, M. M., & Bernt, F. M.
Article Title: Disease chronicity and quality of care in hospital readmissions
Journal Title: *Journal for Healthcare Quality*
Volume (Issue): 19(2)   **Year:** 1997   **Pages:** 33–36

Summary: The study described in this article examined disease chronicity and quality of care and their relationship to hospital readmissions during a 3-month period. Results showed that readmissions due to disease chronicity were significantly more prevalent than for other categories. Illnesses, including pulmonary disease, heart failure, and cancer, ranked as leading causes for readmission, whereas readmissions due to quality of care or complications most often resulted from a previous admission for surgery. This study's finding demonstrate that using readmission rates alone as indicators of poor care can be misleading.

Author(s): Moore, K., Lynn, M. R., McMillen, B. J., & Evans, S.
Article Title: Implementation of the ANA report card
Journal Title: *Journal of Nursing Administration*
Volume (Issue): 29(6)   **Year:** 1999 (June)   **Pages:** 48–54

Summary: A major challenge in health care today is measuring the quality of care. To explore nursing's contribution to patients in acute care settings, the ANA commissioned the development of the "Nursing Report Card." This study explored whether these report card indicators capture quality care. The convenience sample comprised 1500 patients and 300 nurses from 16 units at an academic medical center. Using regression analysis, the most consistent predictor of outcome indicators was the percentage of registered nurses (RNs) of the total staff.

Author(s): Olt, F., Wilson, D., Ron, A., & Soffel, D.
Article Title: Quality improvement through review of inpatient deaths
Journal Title: *Journal for Healthcare Quality*
Volume (Issue): 19(1)   **Year:** 1997   **Pages:** 12–18

Summary: Emphasis on hospital mortality as a monitoring tool has raised concerns about the validity of mortality rates as a measure of quality care. An in-depth review of all mortalities at Beth Israel Medical Center, New York, NY, was conducted from 1988 through 1993. Clinical issues identified from chart review were referred for departmental physician peer review, and quarterly reports of trends and issues were disseminated to all levels of the institution. Mortality rates declined 21% over the 6 years, from 3.3 to 2.6% of all discharges. Clinical quality issues were identified in less than 3% of all mortalities. The majority of problems were related to delays and appropriateness of treatment (57% of quality issues). The review program identified specific hospital processes for improvement, and, more importantly, created a "watchful concern" about quality-of-care issues throughout the hospital.

Author(s): Redmond, G., & Sorrell, J.
Article Title: Studying patient satisfaction: Patient voices of quality
Journal Title: *Outcomes Management for Nursing Practice*
Volume (Issue): 3(2)   **Year:** 1999   **Pages:** 667–672

Summary: The purpose of this qualitative research study was to describe the lived experience and satisfaction of 20 patients after discharge from two acute care rural hospitals. Issues involved in measuring patient satisfaction are discussed in this article. Results of the research are discussed within the themes of (1) knowledgeable watchfulness, (2) thoughtful presencing, and (3) hospital: home and homeless. One pattern, nursing as a bridge, was found throughout the interviews. The authors recommend incorporating qualitative components in the study of patient satisfaction to capture the subtle, invisible ways that nursing interventions can enhance patient satisfaction with the quality of health care.

Author(s): Reed, L., Blegen, M. A., & Goode, C. S.
Article Title: Adverse patient occurrences as a measure of nursing care quality
Journal Title: *Journal of Nursing Administration*
Volume (Issue): 28(5)   **Year:** 1998 (May)   **Pages:** 62–69

Summary: The purpose of this study was to describe relationships among adverse patient occurrences aggregated at the unit level of measurement. A correlational design was used to examine and describe patterns of relationships among inpatient units in a tertiary care hospital. The results demonstrated positive correlations between medication error rates and patient falls; these adverse occurrences correlated negatively with pressure ulcers, infections, patient complaints, and death. Pressure ulcers, infections, patient complaints, and death intercorrelated positively and also related positively to patient acuity levels. When patient acuity was taken into account, these adverse outcomes appeared to indicate some common underlying characteristic of the units, such as quality of nursing care. This study suggests a relationship between the adverse occurrences that were correlated (pressure ulcers, patient complaints, infection, and death) and the severity of patient illness. Medication error rates and patient fall rates were not correlated with patient acuity and are more likely to indicate quality of nursing care across all types of units.

Author(s): Wakefield, D. S., Hendryx, M. S., Uden-Holman, T., Couch, R., & Helms, C. M.
Article Title: Comparing providers' performance: Problems in making the "report card" analogy fit
Journal Title: *Journal for Healthcare Quality: Promoting Excellence in Healthcare*
Volume (Issue): 18(6)   **Year:** 1996 (November/December) **Pages:** 4–10

Summary: This article examines the applicability of a report card strategy as a means of differentiating among providers on the basis of performance. Thirty-one rural, rural referral, and urban acute care hospitals in the Midwest participated in the study. The reported nosocomial infection rates for different types of nursing units and different hospital groups varied substantially. Likewise, there was marked variation in the nosocomial infection surveillance practices at the hospitals, which were found to explain some of the variation in reported nosocomial infection rates for specific types of nursing units and nosocomial infections. The study concluded that differences in data collection processes may result in incorrect conclusions about differences in the quality of care provided by various providers.

Methods of Quality Measurement (N = 7)

Author(s): Alexander, G. L., & Stone, T. T.
Article Title: System review: A method for investigating medical errors in healthcare settings
Journal Title: *Nursing Case Management*
Volume (Issue): 5(5)   **Year:** 2000 (September/October)   **Pages:** 202–213

Summary: System analysis is a process of evaluating objectives, resources, structure, and design of businesses. System analysis can be used by leaders to collaboratively identify breakthrough opportunities to improve system processes. In health care systems, system analysis can be used to review medical errors (system occurrences) that may place patients at risk for injury, disability, and/or death. This study utilizes a case management approach to identify medical errors. Using an interdisciplinary approach, a System Review Team was developed to identify trends in system occurrences, facilitate communication, and enhance the quality of patient care by reducing medical errors.

Author(s): Barton, A. J., Danek, G., Johns, P., & Coons, M.
Article Title: Improving patient outcomes through CQI: Vascular access planning
Journal Title: *Journal of Nursing Care Quality*
Volume (Issue): 13(2)   **Year:** 1998 (December)   **Pages:** 77–85

Summary: This article reports the use of the continuous quality improvement (CQI) process to improve patient outcomes. The FADE method (focus, analyze, develop, and execute) was used to focus on vascular access planning, analyze data concerning intravenous (IV) therapy, develop a vascular access planning algorithm, and execute implementation of the algorithm. An evaluation study revealed that patients whose vascular access planning was consistent with the algorithm reported fewer IVs, less difficulty starting IVs, and less stress; waited significantly less time until central venous line (CVL) placement (for those who received CVLs); and had significantly shorter lengths of stay.

Author(s): Brickman, R., Axelrod, R., Roberson, D., & Flanagan, C.
Article Title: Clinical process improvement as a means of facilitating health care system integration
Journal Title: *Joint Commission Journal on Quality Improvement*
Volume (Issue): 24(3)   **Year:** 1998 (March)   **Pages:** 143–153

Summary: The Sentara Health System created a team responsible for coordinating clinical process improvement activities across its hospitals and ambulatory physician sites. A standardized approach aimed at coordinating care across sites was the cornerstone of these activities. Significant improvement in patient outcomes and a concomitant decrease in costs of care were accomplished for multiple diseases and procedures. These projects uncovered unanticipated barriers to implementing improvement projects in a complex health care system, which make implementing these activities far more difficult than for an individual hospital with its medical staff. Standardization of care practices, policies, and procedures is considerably enhanced by coordinating these activities across the entire system.

Author(s): Harmon, R. L., Sheehy, L. M., & Davis, D. M.
Article Title: The utility of external performance measurement tools in program evaluation . . . Presented, in part, at the annual meeting of the American Academy of Physical Medicine and Rehabilitation in Chicago in October 1996
Journal Title: *Rehabilitation Nursing*
Volume (Issue): 23(1)   **Year:** 1998 (January/February)   **Pages:** 8–11, 56

Summary: Many rehabilitation hospitals use formal measurement tools to evaluate program performance. The Functional Independence Measure instrument through the Uniform Data System for Medical Rehabilitation (UDS MR) provides information that allows an institution to compare its level of performance to those of other facilities. To assess whether joining UDS MR, along with an institution's CQI efforts, could be associated with improved program performance, the records of a rehabilitation hospital's internal inpatient Program Evaluation System (PES) were reviewed for 6 fiscal years (1990 to 1995). Quality improvement efforts during 1995 (during which a 51% improvement in length of stay efficiency was noted) included education for staff, feedback on team performance, and efforts to formulate clinical pathways. Although external measures of performance do not have a direct effect on quality improvement, they could help to identify areas of potential improvement that might not be appreciated when internal assessment systems are used alone.

Author(s): Pearson, J. L., Lee, J. L., Chang, B. L., Elliott, M., Kahn, K. L., & Rubenstein, L. V.
Article Title: Structured implicit review: A new method for monitoring nursing care quality
Journal Title: *Medical Care*
Volume (Issue): 38(11)   **Year:** 2000 (November)   **Pages:** 1074–1091

Summary: The objective of this study was to develop and evaluate nurse structured implicit review (SIR) methods. Scales reflecting domains of nursing process were developed and tested using a randomly selected sample of medical records from 297 acute care hospitals in five states. Data from the RNAD-HCFA Prospective Payment System study was used for elderly Medicare inpatient subjects having either CHF ($n = 291$) or stroke ($n = 283$). It was concluded that nurse peer review with SIR has adequate inter-rater and excellent scale reliabilities and can be a valuable tool for assessing nurse performance.

Author(s): Schell, J. A., Bynum, C. G., Lynan, K. L., & Shaul, B.
Article Title: Survival analysis in quality improvement: The diabetic kidney disease project extrapolation group estimates
Journal Title: *Journal for Healthcare Quality*
Volume (Issue): 22(4)   **Year:** 2000   **Pages:** 37–44

Summary: Survival analysis is used in a wide variety of research settings to maximize the information extracted from a group of timed observations.

Measures employed in CQI efforts often involve such observations. Yet to date, survival analysis has not been widely used to guide CQI efforts. This article presents the features of survival analysis that are most applicable to CQI efforts and illustrates the application of these techniques to a quality improvement project focused on diabetic kidney disease. Results are compared with those from a "standard" analysis. The interpretation of results is discussed in the context of constraints typical of CQI efforts. The article concludes with a recommendation for broader application of this valuable analytic methodology.

Author(s): Schwab, R. A., DelSorbo, S. M., Cunningham, M. R., Craven, K., & Watson, W. A.
Article Title: Using statistical process control to demonstrate the effect of operational interventions on quality indicators in the emergency department
Journal Title: *Journal for Healthcare Quality*
Volume (Issue): 21(4)   **Year:** 1999   **Pages:** 38–41

Summary: This articles describes the development, implementation, and evaluation of a CQI program in the emergency department (ED) of a large urban county teaching hospital that serves as a level I trauma center. Statistical process control methodology was used to assess the effects of Clinical Operations Interventions on numbers of patients who leave without being seen by a physician (LWBS), an indication of patient dissatisfaction. Pre- and postintervention census and LWBs data were retrieved from a computerized data base already in use, and demonstrated a downward trend following implementation.

Case Management/Clinical Pathways (N = 13)

Author(s): Anderson-Loftin, W., Wood, D., & Whitfield, L.
Article Title: A case study of nursing case management in a rural hospital
Journal Title: *Nursing Administration Quarterly*
Volume (Issue): 19(3)   **Year:** 1995 (Spring)   **Pages:** 33–40

Summary: This article describes the process of implementing a New England model of case management in a rural hospital and the modifications necessary in adapting an urban model to a rural setting. Nursing case management at this institution has been associated with a decrease in the length of stay by 1.7 days for an estimated cost savings of $65,932 for the 16-month study period. Case management has also been instrumental in improving quality of care through a program of continuous quality improvement and in redesigning the RN role. The vision for the future is to extend the nurse–case manager role outside the hospital walls to the community in a collaborative plan that would bill nursing services through physicians' offices.

Author(s): Arford, P. H., & Allred, C. A.
Article Title: Value = quality + cost
Journal Title: *Journal of Nursing Administration*
Volume (Issue): 25(9)   **Year:** 1995 (September)   **Pages:** 64–69

Summary: The goal of this study was the development of a quality index to allow a quantifiable synthesis of selected patient care outcomes and service costs. Development of the quality index took place in the context of a larger project designed to determine the effects of nursing case management on the efficiency and effectiveness of patient care. The cost-effectiveness or value of case management was calculated by dividing the average cost per patient by the respective quality index score. Case management in the moderately uncertain practice environment achieved desired patient care outcomes at a significantly lower cost and at a significantly higher level of quality than in either the low or high uncertainty environments.

Author(s): Aspling, D. L., & Lagoe, R. J.
Article Title: Development and implementation of a program to reduce hospital stays and manage resources on a community-wide basis
Journal Title: *Nursing Administration Quarterly*
Volume (Issue): 20(1)   **Year:** 1995 (Fall)   **Pages:** 1–11

Summary: The study describes an effort to reduce hospital stays and limit the use of expensive resources in the metropolitan area of Syracuse, New York. The program included the implementation of clinical pathways for a number of surgical procedures and medical diagnoses. The effort involved the identification of specific resource variables in a wide range of clinical disciplines. The program was important because it focused on cooperative efforts at length of stay and resource reduction by the staffs of all of the hospitals within a common service area.

Author(s): Ayestas, A. L. S., Diaz, E., & Kirtland, S.
Article Title: Clinical pathways: Improving patient education and influencing readmission rates
Journal Title: *Journal for Healthcare Quality*
Volume (Issue): 17(6) **Year:** 1995 (November/December) **Pages:** 17–25, 47

Summary: Clinical pathways have long been used as a mechanism for implementing a managed care delivery system. They have been effective in highlighting lengths of stay, outcome variances, and systems problems. Clinical pathways play an important part in enhancing quality improvement activities, especially in accordance with the standards of the Joint Commission on Accreditation of Healthcare Organizations (JCAHO). This article addresses benefits of clinical pathways in general, and benefits at the authors' facility in particular, specifically, a clinical pathway's effectiveness in influencing readmissions for patients with atrial fibrillation.

Author(s): Bailey, D. A., Litaker, D. G., & Mion, L. C.
Article Title: Developing better critical paths in healthcare: Combining 'best practice' and the quantitative approach
Journal Title: *Journal of Nursing Administration*
Volume (Issue): 28(7/8) **Year:** 1998 (July/August) **Pages:** 21–26

Summary: Critical paths are tools to manage health care delivery and ensure favorable patient outcomes. Unfortunately, many of these paths are not evaluated or revised after their initial development. One potential problem faced by nursing managers is that critical paths may lose relevance in a rapidly changing health care environment. The authors suggest one strategy to strengthen existing critical paths in a way that is responsive to these changes.

Author(s): Chiverton, P., Tortoretti, D., LaForest, M., & Walker, P. H.
Article Title: Bridging the gap between psychiatric hospitalization and community care: Cost and quality outcomes
Journal Title: *Journal of the American Psychiatric Nurses Association*
Volume (Issue): 5(2) **Year:** 1999 (April) **Pages:** 46–53

Summary: The objectives of this study were to (a) investigate differences in quality indicators for patients receiving case management services, (b) measure satisfaction of patients enrolled in the case management intervention, and (c) reduce costs related to high utilization of services as a result of recidivism and rehospitalization. Inpatients were randomly assigned to either an intervention ($n = 121$) or control ($n = 122$) group. The intervention group received transitional case management services, and the control group received traditional care. No differences were found between the two groups on the Beck Depression Inventory or the Mini-Mental Status Examination. Ninety-six percent of the patients and 95% of their caregivers were very pleased with the case management intervention. Fewer patients in the intervention group (9 versus 16 in the control group) were readmitted to the hospital over the course of the project. Similarly, only 1 patient in the intervention group versus 18 patients in the control group used the ED. Even considering the cost of providing case management services, an overall savings of $175, 375 occurred for the intervention group. Transitional case management services maintained quality and reduced costs with a high level of consumer satisfaction.

Author(s): Crawley, W. D., & Till, A. H.
Article Title: Case management: More population-based data
Journal Title: *Clinical Nurse Specialist*
Volume (Issue): 9(2) **Year:** 1995 **Pages:** 116–120

Summary: A pilot project conducted in a 540-bed teaching hospital reveals more population-based data related to nursing case management, a system of patient care that promotes cost containment and ensures quality outcomes. Positive outcomes were demonstrated in quality of care, patient satisfaction, staff satisfaction, length of stay, and cost.

Author(s): Grant, P. H., Campbell, L. L., & Gautney, L. J.
Article Title: Implementing case management and developing clinical pathways
Journal Title: *Journal for Healthcare Quality*
Volume (Issue): 17(6) **Year:** 1995 (November/December) **Pages:** 10–16

Summary: Efforts to implement case management and, subsequently, to develop critical paths at Birmingham Baptist Medical Center Montclair in Birmingham, Alabama, began in the late 1980s. Under the case management system, RNs using the CareMap system manage the care of 60 to 80% of the medical center's patients. Those patients whose care did not follow a map are managed by nurse–case managers. Patients who do not meet the identified goals for care require a collaborative effort from all the health care professionals associated with their care. Since the inception of the case management program, Montclair has made significant strides in decreasing the cost per discharge, decreasing the variable cost per case, and improving quality outcomes for designated case types.

Author(s): Ireson, C. L.
Article Title: Critical pathways: Effectiveness in achieving patient outcomes
Journal Title: *Journal of Nursing Administration*
Volume (Issue): 27(6) **Year:** 1997 (June) **Pages:** 16–23

Summary: Refining the clinical care process to produce high-quality patient outcomes is becoming increasingly important as health care administrators strive for success in a mature managed care environment. This study examines the effect of structuring interventions and the evaluation of patient response, inherent in the critical pathway process, on clinical, length-of-hospital-stay, and financial patient outcomes. This study differs from previous critical pathway trials in that an objective measure of quality was used and the critical pathways were not introduced concurrently with a case management delivery model. The results show that critical pathways may be a significant determinant of improved quality in a managed care environment. The findings also suggest ways to improve nursing practice, nursing education, and nursing informatics.

Author(s): Little, A. B., & Whipple, T. W.
Article Title: Clinical pathway implementation in the acute care hospital setting
Journal Title: *Journal of Nursing Care Quality*
Volume (Issue): 11(2) **Year:** 1996 (December) **Pages:** 54–61

Summary: A study was conducted to assess the current status of clinical path implementation for acute care cases and to explore implementation issues related to defining discharge outcomes and measuring variances in clinical paths. Results indicated that documentation, identification of critical indicators and discharge outcomes, and variance detection and correction are three core issues that must be addressed by institutions that implement clinical paths. A discussion of each of these areas is provided.

Author(s): Lynn, M. R., & Kelley, B.
Article Title: Effects of case management on the nursing context—Perceived quality of care, work satisfaction, and control over practice
Journal Title: *Image—The Journal of Nursing Scholarship*
Volume (Issue): 29(3) **Year:** 1997 **Pages:** 237–241

Summary: The purpose of this prospective quasi-experimental study was to examine the effects of case management on the context of nursing practice-perceived quality of care delivered, work satisfaction, and control over nursing practice. Sampled were nurses on four units at one community hospital where patients with DRG 107 (Coronary Artery Bypass Graft [CABG], with no cardiac catheterization) were traditionally hospitalized. RNs on these units completed quality of care, satisfaction, and practice control scales before and 1 year after implementation. Significant positive differences were found in nurses' perceived ability to develop relationships with patients, ability to be therapeutic, and support for good care from the institutional structure and administration. A significant decrease in nurses' satisfaction with their pay and other rewards as well as respect from colleagues was found. Case managers were found to have significantly increased perceptions of control over their practice. Additionally, case managers were more satisfied with the administration, the respect they received, and their pay and rewards in the institution. Most strikingly, case managers perceived themselves to have more control over their practice. Negative effects of the program were a decrease in satisfaction with the pay and rewards by the staff who were not case managers.

Author(s): Thompson, D. G., & Maringer, M.
Article Title: Using case management to improve care delivery in the NICU
Journal Title: *MCN, American Journal of Maternal Child Nursing*
Volume (Issue): 20(5) **Year:** 1995 **Pages:** 257–260

Summary: A comparison study demonstrates that length of stay and average costs decrease for high-risk infants, and that quality of care is strengthened.

Author(s): Waters, J. B., Wolff, R. S., Blansfield, J., LaMorte, W. W., Millham, F. H., & Hirsch, E. F.
Article Title: Development and implementation of clinical pathways for the management of four trauma diagnoses
Journal Title: *Journal for Healthcare Quality*
Volume (Issue): 21(3)   **Year:** 1999   **Pages:** 4–11

Summary: This article deals with the process by which four diagnoses (closed head injury, penetrating wound to the abdomen, chest, and extremity) were identified and the pathways designed, implemented, and evaluated. Upon implementation of these pathways, appropriate nonoperative, single-system, short-stay trauma patients were enrolled in them. Preliminary data demonstrate a significant decrease in resource utilization following implementation of the pathways, without an adverse impact on readmission rates, length of stay, or mortality.

Patient Safety (N = 9)

Author(s): Alcee, D.
Article Title: The experience of a community hospital in quantifying and reducing patient falls
Journal Title: *Journal of Nursing Care Quality*
Volume (Issue): 14(3)   **Year:** 2000 (April)   **Pages:** 43–53

Summary: A retrospective review of patient falls in a 248-bed acute care community hospital was conducted to quantify the number of patient falls and identify what factors resulted in these falls. The author reports these results and describes specific measures that were implemented in an attempt to reduce the number of falls in the organization.

Author(s): Bankert, K., Daughtridge, S., Meehan, M., & Colburn, L.
Article Title: The application of collaborative benchmarking to the prevention and treatment of pressure ulcers
Journal Title: *Advances in Wound Care: The Journal for Prevention & Healing*
Volume (Issue): 9(2)   **Year:** 1996 (March/April)   **Pages:** 21–29

Summary: In the spring of 1995, 42 hospitals participated in a collaborative benchmarking study on the prevention and treatment of pressure ulcers. The study resulted in the discovery of 54 best practices that, taken together, provide a blueprint for successful actions and processes that can easily be adapted to individual institutional needs. An important finding of this benchmarking study showed that the four hospitals with lowest risk-adjusted, hospital-acquired prevalence rates were the same four hospitals identified as benchmarks in at least four other critical success factors. During the study, representatives were exposed not only to the practices of care delivered at other hospitals, but also to the rationale, limitations, and success of those practices. This understanding, coupled with the best practices, has helped representatives to improve their facilities' pressure ulcer programs.

Author(s): Carey, R., & Teeters, J.
Article Title: CQI case study: Reducing medication errors
Journal Title: *The Joint Commission Journal on Quality Improvement*
Volume (Issue): 21(5)   **Year:** 1995   **Pages:** 233–237

Summary: This article describes how one hospital formed a CQI team and used statistical process control tools to assess efforts to reduce medication errors. The team worked with nursing staff to develop an IV training module for nurses that effectively decreased the average number of errors per month. The article illustrates the effective use of a run chart, a Pareto chart, and tow types of control charts to identify an opportunity for improvement, develop an improvement strategy, and measure the effectiveness of the intervention.

Author(s): Hopkins, B., Hanlon, M., Yauk, S., Sykes, S., & Rose, T.
Article Title: Reducing nosocomial pressure ulcers
Journal Title: *Journal of Nursing Care Quality*
Volume (Issue): 14(3)   **Year:** 2000 (April)   **Pages:** 28–36

Summary: In 1996, a nursing committee at an acute care facility organized the first pressure ulcer point prevalence survey for that hospital. In 1996, hospital-acquired pressure ulcers were 90% of the predicted prevalence rate; in 1997, the rate dropped to 59% of the predicted prevalence, and in 1998, to 53% of the predicted prevalence. The severity index decreased markedly from 291 (1996) to 98 (1997) and then to 62 (1998). These improvements are attributed to the purposeful addition of multidimensional interventions, including best practices and research-based protocols, to prevent and treat nosocomial pressure ulcers.

Author(s): Huda, A., & Wise, L. C.
Article Title: Evolution of compliance within a fall prevention program
Journal Title: *Journal of Nursing Care Quality*
Volume (Issue): 12(3)   **Year:** 1998 (February)   **Pages:** 55–63

Summary: When evaluating the effectiveness of a fall prevention program, it is useful to first determine whether the program is being uniformly administered. Members of a medical-surgical unit's Quality Assurance/Product Improvement Team studied both processes as well as outcomes over a 2-year implementation of a fall prevention program. They discovered that initial attempts at implementation underestimated the quantity of resources necessary to ensure full implementation of the program. This article chronicles the series of audits and program modifications that eventually brought success to this unit.

Author(s): Minnick, A. F., Mion, L. C., Leipzig, R., Lamb, K., & Palmer, R. M.
Article Title: Prevalence and patterns of physical restraint use in the acute care setting
Journal Title: *Journal of Nursing Administration*
Volume (Issue): 28(11)   **Year:** 1998 (November)   **Pages:** 19–22

Summary: The results of this three-site, interdisciplinary, prospective incidence study reveal new patterns in the rationale and types of restraints used. Observational surveys were carried out in three tertiary, urban, teaching, referral centers located in Midwestern states. More than 49,000 observations were collected on 18 randomly selected days across all nonemergency, nonpsychiatric, nonobstetric units across the three facilities revealed a 5.8% overall rate of restraint use. Although differences in usage rates were noted across institutions, rates were consistently higher in intensive care units (ICUs).

Author(s): Stetler, C. B., Morsi, D., & Burns, M.
Article Title: Physical and emotional patient safety: A different look at nursing-sensitive outcomes
Journal Title: *Outcomes Management for Nursing Practice*
Volume (Issue): 4(4)   **Year:** 2000 (October/December)   **Pages:** 159–166

Summary: Data on nursing-sensitive outcomes, beyond traditional isolated indicators such as pressure ulcers, are often unavailable for nurses to evaluate the overall quality of their care. This article describes a quality improvement effort to provide nurses with both a positive and a negative patient outcomes score. The approach can make visible the often invisible role of nurses in the growing field of patient safety.

Author(s): Swauger, K. C., & Tomlin, C. C.
Article Title: Moving toward restraint-free patient care
Journal Title: *Journal of Nursing Administration*
Volume (Issue): 30(6) **Year:** 2000 (June) **Pages:** 325–329

Summary: This article describes an empirically based restraint reduction program in an urban, tertiary referral center. *Reducing Restraints: Individualized Approaches to Behavior* published by Geriatric Research and training Center was modified and implemented by a "restraint team" chartered for the specific purpose of restraint reduction. Chart review of all restrained patients and all patients who required a restraint consult indicated that restraints were reduced by 60%, and that restraints applied were least restrictive.

Author(s): Zollo, M. B., Gostisha, M. L., Berens, R. J., Schmidt, J. E., & Weigle, C. G. M.
Article Title: Altered skin integrity in children admitted to a pediatric intensive care unit
Journal Title: *Journal of Nursing Care Quality*
Volume (Issue): 11(2) **Year:** 1996 (December) **Pages:** 62–67

Summary: As part of a quality improvement study, the incidence and severity of altered skin integrity in a tertiary pediatric intensive care unit (PICU) were investigated in an attempt to identify contributing risk factors. Demographic, severity of illness, and practice variables were collected on 271 of 357 admissions during an 18-week period. Data were analyzed from the date of PICU admission until a change in skin integrity occurred or until PICU discharge. Altered skin integrity occurred in 26% of admissions; 7% of the cases had skin breakdown. By multivariate analysis, only the Pediatric Risk of Mortality Score and white race were associated with altered skin integrity.

Pain and Pain Management (N = 12)

Author(s): Bergh, I., & Sjostrom, B.

Article Title: A comparative study of nurses' and elderly patients' ratings of pain and pain tolerance

Journal Title: *Journal of Gerontological Nursing*

Volume (Issue): 25(5)   **Year:** 1999 (May)   **Pages:** 30–42

Summary: Nurses tend to overestimate mild pain and underestimate severe pain. The tendency to underestimate severe pain increased with the severity marked by patients on the Visual Analogue Scale. There was a significant difference in ratings of pain tolerance (eg, when pain should be treated) between nurses and patients. The nurses with training higher than basic nursing education tend to assess the patients' experiences of pain more correctly than those without additional training. For patients who reported that they had not encountered pain prior to hospitalization, the nurses' ratings of pain showed a higher agreement than for those who reported that they had encountered pain before being hospitalized.

Author(s): Bookbinder, M., Coyle, N., Kiss, M., Goldstein, M. L., Holritz, K., Thaler, H., Gianella, A., Derby, S., Brown, M., Racolin, A., Ho, M. N., & Portenoy, R. K.

Article Title: Implementing national standards for cancer pain management: Program model and evaluation

Journal Title: *Journal of Pain & Symptom Management*

Volume (Issue): 12(6)   **Year:** 1996 (December)   **Pages:** 334–347

Summary: The purpose of this quasi-experimental (pre- and posttest) study was to test a model pain management program (PMP) to implement the American Pain Society (APS) quality assurance standards for the management of acute and chronic cancer pain using a CQI approach. The sample consisted of 1210 nurse responses and 698 interviews of patients with pain during hospitalization at a major urban cancer center. The PMP provided a structure (standards), educational opportunities, and training in CQI methods. Outcome measures included a patient evaluation questionnaire and concerns checklist; nurse knowledge, attitude, and barriers questionnaire; and focus groups to identify areas needing improvement. Significant improvements were found in patients' satisfaction, nurses' knowledge and attitude scores, and reductions in nurses' perceptions of barriers. Focus groups revealed the need for improved communication among disciplines about pain and better assessment of patients unable to self-report. The program met its goal of implementing the APS standards, educating nurses, identifying "system" problems, and improving overall patient satisfaction.

Author(s): Buchanan, L., Voigtman, J., & Mills, H.

Article Title: Implementing the Agency for Health Care Policy and Research Pain Management Pediatric Guideline in a multicultural practice setting

Journal Title: *Journal of Nursing Care Quality*

Volume (Issue): 11(3)   **Year:** 1997 (February)   **Pages:** 23–35

Summary: This article describes the implementation, monitoring, and evaluation of a clinical practice guideline for managing pediatric patient pain. The standard of care used was the Agency for Health Care Policy and Research (AHCPR) acute pain management guideline. It was used to assess current levels of care and to make recommendations for improvements. Information was gathered from a sample of 240 pediatric patients aged 1 week to 14 years. Recommendations for improving care are given. The guideline was found to be clinically useful as a general standard of care, but more work needs to be done to individualize care for specific populations, age groups, and cultures.

Author(s): Caswell, D. R., Williams, J. P., Vallejo, M., Zaroda, T., McNair, N., Keckeisen, M., Yale, C., & Cryer, H.G.
Article Title: Improving pain management in critical care
Journal Title: *Journal on Quality Improvement*
Volume (Issue): 22(10) **Year:** 1996 **Pages:** 702–712

Summary: One year after implementation of a practice guideline and a re-education effort that still continues, ICU patients report markedly less pain.

Author(s): Calvin, A., Becker, H., Biering, P., & Grobe, S.
Article Title: Measuring patient opinion of pain management
Journal Title: *Journal of Pain & Symptom Management*
Volume (Issue): 18(1) **Year:** 1999 (July) **Pages:** 17–26

Summary: Pain management has been increasingly recognized as an important indicator of quality patient care. In this article, we describe the development of a measure of patients' perception of pain management. Based on the American Pain Society's guidelines, the six-item Patient Opinion of Pain Management (POPM) scale demonstrated promising internal consistency, reliability, and validity in a sample of 241 patients from 11 hospitals. The POPM is discussed in the context of previous research on the assessment of pain management.

Author(s): Celia, B.
Article Title: Age and gender differences in pain management following coronary artery bypass surgery
Journal Title: *Journal of Gerontological Nursing*
Volume (Issue): 26(5) **Year:** 2000 (May) **Pages:** 7–13

Summary: Undermedication of patients' pain by nurses persists despite pain management advances over the past 20 years. Nurses' assessment of patients' pain has been identified as problematic because of the lack of use of a pain rating scale. Elderly individuals and women are particularly vulnerable to undermedication of pain, possibly because of misconceptions that persist. Nurses would benefit from educational programs related to pain management of all groups regardless of culture, gender, and age.

Author(s): Dalton, J.A., Blau, W., Lindley, C., Carlson, J., Youngblood, R., & Greer, S. M.
Article Title: Changing acute pain management to improve patient outcomes: An educational approach
Journal Title: *Journal of Pain & Symptom Management*
Volume (Issue): 17(4) **Year:** 1999 (April) **Pages:** 277–287

Summary: This article describes the development and implementation of an education program for nurses, physicians, and pharmacists in six community hospitals. Program content addressing the use of CQI teams, detailed pain histories, application of algorithms, and dose calculation is described; direct and indirect outcome measures are reviewed. Six months after the program, all three experimental sites reported use of the AHCPR Guidelines in practice. Nurses reported that assessment and documentation of patients' duration of pain were perceived to be the most important caregiver behaviors providing benefit to patients: Across all respondents' reports of regularly performed activities, the activity performed by the largest proportion was assessing and documenting pain using a 0 to 10 rating scale.

Author(s): Paice, J., Mahon, S. M., & Faut-Callahan, M.
Article Title: Pain control in hospitalized postsurgical patients
Journal Title: *MEDSURG Nursing*
Volume (Issue): 4(5)   Year: 1995   Pages: 367–372

Summary: The purpose of this study was to describe the pain experience of 100 randomly selected postsurgical patients; identify discrepancies between physician, nurse, and patient reports of pain intensity; and characterize the documentation of patients' pain experiences within the hospital record.

Author(s): Sayers, M., Marando, R., Fisher, S., Aquila, A., Morrison, B., & Dailey, T.
Article Title: No need for pain
Journal Title: *Journal for Healthcare Quality*
Volume (Issue): 22(3)   Year: 2000 (May/June)   Pages: 10–14

Summary: This article describes a collaborative quality improvement initiative designed to promote effective pain management. Data were collected through staff evaluations; patient satisfaction studies; measurement of the effectiveness of analgesic care; frequency of meperidine usage and IM injections; and measurement of staff knowledge of pain management, and their comfort level with pain management. Positive outcomes reported include a significant increase ($p = .01$) in physicians and nurses discussing with their patients the importance of managing their pain, development of processes for documenting pain as the fifth vital sign, and a 26% decrease in the use of meperidine.

Author(s): Sherwood, G., Adams-McNeill, J., Starck, P. L., Nieto, B., & Thompson, C. J.
Article Title: Qualitative assessment of hospitalized patients' satisfaction with pain management
Journal Title: *Research in Nursing & Health*
Volume (Issue): 23(6)   Year: 2000 (December)   Pages: 486–495

Summary: This descriptive, qualitative study was designed to examine the acute pain experience of hospitalized patients to address gaps and clarify how pain and its management influenced patients to report satisfaction or dissatisfaction. The sample comprised 241 adult patients who were hospitalized for at least 24 hours, postsurgical or diagnosed with a painful condition. Data for the descriptive qualitative portion of the study came from three open-ended questions that were part of a 16-item survey, the American Pain Society Patient Outcome Questionnaire—Modified. The study contributes to our understanding of patient responses to pain through a typology of factors that influences levels of satisfaction. It became clear that even though patients expressed disbelief of pain myths on the written questionnaire, their behaviors at the time of pain were based on these beliefs. Interview responses suggest that patient education is needed to overcome lack of knowledge, fear of addiction, side effects, and unrealistic concerns about taking pain medications and to reduce tendencies to suffer in silence.

Author(s): Starck, P. L., Adams, J., Sherwood, G., & Thompson, C.
Article Title: Development of a pain management report card for an acute care setting
Journal Title: *Advanced Practice Nursing Quarterly*
Volume (Issue): 3(2)   **Year:** 1997 (Fall)   **Pages:** 57–63

Summary: The article describes a pain management report card developed as a result of a study on pain satisfaction. The report card presented the actual results of the study and compared them with the institution's predetermined goals. Comparison items included adherence to national pain guidelines for pain management, various measures of the pain experience, and satisfaction with nurse and physician caregivers related to pain management. Recommendations were made to the institution based on the findings.

Author(s): Stratton, L.
Article Title: Evaluating the effectiveness of a hospital's pain management program
Journal Title: *Journal of Nursing Care Quality*
Volume (Issue): 13(4)   **Year:** 1999 (April)   **Pages:** 8–18

Summary: Nationally, the focus on facilities providing effective pain management has increased, yet no funds have been allocated to pain management programs. The article describes a 3-year study whose purpose was to evaluate the effect on nurses' attitudes and behavior of the institution of a multifaceted, low-cost hospital pain management program. The program utilized various instructional methods and implementation of policies, procedures, and documentation protocols. Nurses were surveyed before and after the pain management program using the 39-item Nurses' Knowledge and Attitudes Survey. Results demonstrated a statistically significant increase between pretest and posttest scores.

Care Delivery Models (N = 9)

Author(s): Black, E., Weiss, K., Erban, S., & Shulkin, D.
Article Title: Innovations in patient care: Changing clinical practice and improving quality
Journal Title: *The Joint Commission Journal on Quality Improvement*
Volume (Issue): 21(8)   **Year:** 1995   **Pages:** 376–393

Summary: One hospital developed an Innovations in Patient Care (IPC) program, which several other medical centers have duplicated. One study, whose principal investigator was assistant director of emergency medicine, showed that structured, condition-specific (eg, asthma, pharyngitis, lacerations, and isolated closed head injury) quick-sheets improved documentation of clinical findings, resource use, and clinical practice. A study organized by the leadership of surgical nursing revealed that a nursing case management model led to reductions in patient length of stay and increase in nurse satisfaction. IPC programs, which integrate well with initiatives in total quality management (TQM), can be effectively used to change clinical practice and improve the quality and efficiency of patient care.

Author(s): Counsell, S. R., Holder, C. M., Liebenauer, L. L., Palmer, R. M., Fortinsky, R. H., Kresevic, D. M., Quinn, L. M., Allen, K. R., Covinsky, K. E., & Landefeld, C. S.
Article Title: Effects of a multicomponent intervention on functional outcomes and process of care in hospitalized older patients: A randomized controlled trial of acute care for elders (ACE) in a community hospital
Journal Title: *Journal of the American Geriatrics Society*
Volume (Issue): 48(12)   **Year:** 2000 (December)   **Pages:** 1572–1581

Summary: This randomized controlled trial study tested the hypothesis that a multi-component intervention, called Acute Care for Elders (ACE), will improve functional outcomes and the process of care in hospitalized older patients. A total of 531 community-dwelling patients, aged 70 or older, were admitted for an acute medical illness between November 1994 and May 1997. ACE includes a specially designed environment (eg, with carpeting and uncluttered hallways); patient-centered care, including nursing care plans for prevention of disability and rehabilitation; planning for patient discharge to home; and review of medical care to prevent iatrogenic illness. ACE in a community hospital improved the process of care and patient and provider satisfaction without increasing hospital length of stay or costs. A lower frequency of the composite outcome activities of daily living (ADL) decline or nursing home placement may indicate potentially beneficial effects on patient outcomes.

Author(s): Covinsky, K. E., Palmer, R. M., Kresevic, D. M., Kahana, E., Counsell, S. R., Fortinsky, R. H., & Landefeld, C. S.
Article Title: Improving functional outcomes in older patients: Lessons from an acute care for elders unit
Journal Title: *Journal on Quality Improvement*
Volume (Issue): 24(2)   **Year:** 1998   **Pages:** 63–76

Summary: University Hospitals of Cleveland implemented an ACE unit and demonstrated that such a unit improves short-term outcomes and may decrease costs, with long-term benefits still to be determined.

Author(s): Heinemann, D., Lengacher, C. A., VanCott, M. L., Mabe, P., & Swymer, S.
Article Title: Partners in patient care: Measuring the effects on patient satisfaction and other quality indicators
Journal Title: *Nursing Economics*
Volume (Issue): 14(5)   **Year:** 1996 (September–October)   **Pages:** 276–285

Summary: An experimental pretest/posttest design compared pilot and control nursing units in a medical center in southwest Florida to assess the effects of a Partners in Patient Care (PIPC) nursing care delivery model on selected quality of care outcomes—patient satisfaction, patient medication errors, falls, and IV infections. There were no significant differences between units in the number of falls, medication errors, and IV infections. When the ratios of these events to patient days were examined, there was a significant difference between the pilot and control units in the medication error ratio and the fall ratio. The results indicate that the PIPC nursing model has a positive effect on patient satisfaction.

Author(s): Jones, R. A. P., Dougherty, M., & Martin, S.
Article Title: Program evaluation of a unit reengineered for patient-focused care
Journal Title: *Holistic Nursing Practice*
Volume (Issue): 11(3)   **Year:** 1997 (April)   **Pages:** 31–46

Summary: A quasi-experimental research design was used to determine how successful a work redesign project based on the philosophy of patient-focused care was in meeting the established goals of increased multidisciplinary collaboration, improved satisfaction for health care clients and providers, decreased cost of care, and decreased length of stay. Results indicate that multidisciplinary collaboration decreased for all health care providers, especially the health care employee group that underwent a major role revision. Patient and health care provider satisfaction increased. The cost of care was budget neutral as a result of the shift of employee costs from centralized departments to units. Length of stay decreased.

Author(s): Miller, D., Smith, D. J., Brophy, M., Mollman, M., Owen, J., Smith, G., & More, C.
Article Title: Total quality improvement: An example of an effective team
Journal Title: *Journal for Healthcare Quality*
Volume (Issue): 18(1)   **Year:** 1996 (January/February)   **Pages:** 20–23

Summary: TQI advocates that all staff members in an organization develop their own ideas on job improvement about their own specific jobs. This process helps to improve staff performance and to build continually on those improvements. This article describes how the TQI process was used successfully by quality management staff members at a federal medical center to investigate a problem with linen.

Author(s): Nardone, P. L., Markie, J. W., & Tolle S.
Article Title: Evaluating a nursing care delivery model using a quality improvement design
Journal Title: *Journal of Nursing Care Quality*
Volume (Issue): 10(1)   **Year:** 1995   **Pages:** 70–84

Summary: This evaluative study used both quantitative and qualitative methods. Seven principles related to quality were identified and became the driving force behind the changes. Aspects of these changes in care delivery were piloted on a neurologic unit and included implementation of collaborative rounds, a modular structure, role changes, and work redesign. Frequency distribution, questionnaire, focus group, and financial data indicated that there had been improvement in the delivery of care in addition to the financial benefits realized. A considerable amount of the data provided evidence that supported continuing the changes.

Author(s): Nash, M. G., Grant, J. S., & Bartolucci, A. A.
Article Title: Clinical and operational outcomes of a work redesign model
Journal Title: *National Academies of Practice Forum: Issues in Interdisciplinary Care (NAPF)*
Volume (Issue): 2(3)   **Year:** 2000 (July)   **Pages:** 203–210

Summary: This study examined the impact of a work redesign model, Patient Care 2000 (PC2000), on salary costs, patient satisfaction, quality of care, nurse–patient contacts, and quality of employee work life. Data were derived from cost analysis reports, questionnaires, chart reviews, and direct observation. The setting for the study was a major academic health care and tertiary referral center. Participants were patients, RNs, and other hospital employees. The intervention was the PC2000 work redesign model. Outcome measures were salary costs, patient satisfaction scores, hospital-acquired pressure ulcers, nurse–patient contacts, and quality of employee work life scores. There was a significant decrease in salary costs and an increase in nurse–patient contacts, but no differences were found related to other outcome measures. This model may be useful in reducing salary costs and increasing nurse–patient contacts while maintaining pre-implementation levels of other outcomes.

Author(s): Peruzzi, M., Ringer, D., & Tassey, K.
Article Title: A community hospital redesigns care
Journal Title: *Nursing Administration Quarterly*
Volume (Issue): 20(1)   **Year:** 1995 (Fall)   **Pages:** 24–46

Summary: In response to professional and societal forces, Albany Memorial Hospital redesigned patient care services. Funding as a New York State Workforce Demonstration project afforded the organization the resources to study components such as decentralization of services, case management, and reallocation of workers to new or expanded roles. Subsequent changes in skill mix were associated with improved or unchanged quality indicators and satisfaction levels. Cost savings were demonstrated by adjusted labor costs and continue through present housewide use of caremapping. Although the process requires tremendous time and energy, the outcomes clearly justify the investment.

Staff and Staffing (N = 10)

Author(s): Blegen, M. A., & Vaughn, T.
Article Title: A multisite study of nurse staffing and patient occurrences
Journal Title: *Nursing Economics*
Volume (Issue): 16(4) **Year:** 1998 (July–August) **Pages:** 196–203

Summary: The purpose of this study, wherein data were collected from 39 units in 11 hospitals, was to determine the relationship between different levels of nurse staffing and patient outcomes (adverse occurrences). Among the more surprising findings in this study was the nonlinear relationship between the proportion of RNs in the staff mix and medications administration errors (MAEs). As the proportion of RNs on a unit increased from 50 to 85% "the rate of MAEs declined, but as the RN proportion increased from 85 to 100% the rate of MAEs increased." Further investigations are needed to explain this finding.

Author(s): Freer, Y., & Murphy-Black, T.
Article Title: Work rotas and performance levels: Evaluating the effects of twelve hour shifts against eight hour shifts on a neonatal intensive care unit
Journal Title: *Journal of Neonatal Nursing*
Volume (Issue): 1(4) **Year:** 1995 **Pages:** 5–9

Summary: Efficiency drives have led to changes in staffing levels and working rotas, but the resulting effects on provision and quality of care are unclear. A repeated measures study was conducted with staff working in a NICU using self-assessment questionnaires to record quality of care and influencing factors of quality as perceived by them under a 12-hour shift rota as compared to an 8-hour shift rota. The 12-hour rota showed increased levels of satisfaction by caregivers in the provision and overall standard of care.

Author(s): Friedman, C., & Chenoweth, C.
Article Title: A survey of infection control professional staffing patterns at University HealthSystem consortium institutions
Journal Title: *American Journal of Infection Control*
Volume (Issue): 26(3) **Year:** 1998 (June) **Pages:** 239–244

Summary: To provide current benchmarking comparison data for expected staff reductions, a survey of University Health System Consortium members was performed. An infection control professional at each institution was contacted to obtain most of the information. Responses were obtained from 45 University Health System Consortium members (67%). Full-time equivalent ratios were based on the following parameters and compared for the institutions: number of occupied beds (median 137 occupied beds), number of ICU beds (median 28 beds), number of admissions or discharges (median 6686 admissions), number of ambulatory care visits (median 104,426 visits), and case-mix index (median 1.75). Many institutions are using benchmarking comparison data to make decisions regarding staff reductions. This survey provides preliminary data for determining the "best practice" in staffing for infection control departments. More information may be needed to evaluate other factors that affect infection control professionals' workload.

Author(s): Hansen, B. S., & Benitez, D. I.
Article Title: Quantified caring
Journal Title: *Nursing Administration Quarterly*
Volume (Issue): 24(4)   **Year:** 2000 (Summer)   **Pages:** 72–79

Summary: In partnership with a consulting firm, a system was implemented in one hospital that measures and correlates patient satisfaction, quality, and cost in real time. The findings revealed that more staff does not necessarily equal higher patient satisfaction scores. Award-winning hospitals have achieved and sustained patient satisfaction scores above 90% without adding staff by keeping score with real-time data.

Author(s): Knaus, V. L., Felten, S., Burton, S., Fobes, P., & Davis, K.
Article Title: The use of nurse practitioners in the acute care setting
Journal Title: *Journal of Nursing Administration*
Volume (Issue): 27(2)   **Year:** 1997 (February)   **Pages:** 20–27

Summary: A collaborative practice model was initiated in a university hospital to assist resident physicians to coordinate patient care on specialty services. Nurse practitioner (NP) data were collected on daily work activities and categorized as direct care, indirect care, administration, education, and research.

Author(s): Lichtig, L. K., Knauf, R. A., & Milholland, D. K.
Article Title: Some impacts of nursing on acute care hospital outcomes
Journal Title: *Journal of Nursing Administration*
Volume (Issue): 29(2)   **Year:** 1999 (February)   **Pages:** 25–33

Summary: Using data from California and New York, this study tested the feasibility of measuring nurse-sensitive patient outcomes in the acute care hospitals, and examined relationships between these outcomes and nurse staffing. Nurse intensity weights were used to acuity adjust patient data. Both higher nurse staffing and higher proportion of RNs were significantly related to shorter lengths of stay. Lower adverse outcome rates were more consistently related to a higher proportion of RNs.

Author(s): Luther, K. M., & Walsh, K.
Article Title: Moving out of the red zone: Addressing staff allocation to improve patient satisfaction
Journal Title: *Journal on Quality Improvement*
Volume (Issue): 25(7)   **Year:** 1999   **Pages:** 363–368

Summary: When patients hospitalized in August 1997 experienced dissatisfaction with care, the hospital was listening. Each summer, Hermann Hospital (Houston) experienced staffing challenges because of employee vacations. A "zone" system was developed to address staff allocation, which was identified as a factor in deterioration of the hospital's patient satisfaction performance.

Author(s): Minnick, A. F, & Pabst, M. K.
Article Title: Improving the ability to detect the impact of labor on patient outcomes
Journal Title: *Journal of Nursing Administration*
Volume (Issue): 28(12)   **Year:** 1998 (December)   **Pages:** 17–21

Summary: This national study lends support for a previously identified labor assignment phenomena that may contribute to an underestimation of the impact of nursing labor on outcomes if only traditional labor measurement methods are used. Based on staffing data collected from 8 hospitals, 77 units, and representing 596 weeks of assignments, the authors identified a tendency to assign fewer staff members than required to units with high staff quantity requirements, based on patient care needs. Assignment patterns demonstrated "remarkable stability" over the 6- to 8-week study period.

Author(s): Sochalski, J., Estabrooks, C. A., & Humphrey, C. K.
Article Title: Nurse staffing and patient outcomes: Evolution of an international study
Journal Title: *Canadian Journal of Nursing Research*
Volume (Issue): 31(3)   **Year:** 1999 (December)   **Pages:** 69–88

Summary: Industry-wide health sector reforms in the United States, Canada, and Europe have provided a unique opportunity to examine the effects of hospital restructuring on inpatient nursing care and patient outcomes across an array of settings. Seven interdisciplinary research teams—one each in Alberta, British Columbia, England, Germany, Ontario, Scotland, and the United States—have formed an international consortium whose aim is to study the effects of such restructuring. Each site has enrolled large numbers of hospitals and nurses to explicate the role that organization of nursing care, a target of hospital restructuring, plays in differential patient outcomes. The study seeks to understand more fully the influence of both nurse staffing and the nursing practice environment on patient outcomes. The theoretical foundation, study design, and process of developing the study instruments and measures illustrates the process to date are discussed, as well as the feasibility of and opportunities inherent in such an international endeavor.

Author(s): Strzalka, A., & Havens, D. S.
Article Title: Nursing care quality: Comparison of unit-hired, hospital float pool, and agency nurses
Journal Title: *Journal of Nursing Care Quality*
Volume (Issue): 10(4)   **Year:** 1996 (July)   **Pages:** 59–65

Summary: As fiscal constraints and hospital downsizing become driving forces in the health care arena, nurse administrators are challenged to satisfy fluctuating staffing needs while ensuring high-quality care. Hospital in-house nurses and agency nurses are two solutions often used to supplement unit staffing. The article reports a study that examined the quality of care administered on one unit by unit-hired, float pool, and agency nurses through a comparison of the groups' documentation on nine clinical quality indicators. Findings suggested significant differences among the three groups on these indicators. Implications for nurse-administrators are discussed.

Organizational Restructure/Redesign (N = 10)

Author(s): Brett, J. L., Bueno, M., Royal, N., & Kendall-Sengin, K.
Article Title: PRO-ACT II: Integrating utilization management, discharge planning, and nursing care management into the outcomes manager role
Journal Title: *Journal of Nursing Administration*
Volume (Issue): 27(2)   **Year:** 1997 (February)   **Pages:** 37–45

Summary: Building on redesign efforts that created case management, clinical care technicians, support service hosts, and pharmacy technician roles, this redesign focused on integrating case management, utilization management, and discharge planning functions into a new outcomes manager role. The authors describe the process of developing and implementing the new role and outline specific actions that eliminated redundancy and inefficiency. Results of the evaluation of the project are reviewed, including full-time equivalent and salary saving, and employee and physician satisfaction improvements.

Author(s): Bryan, Y. E., Hitchings, K. S., Fuss, M. A., Fox, M. A., Kinneman, M. T., & Young, M. J.
Article Title: Measuring and evaluating hospital restructuring efforts: Eighteen-month follow-up and extension to critical care, part 1
Journal Title: *Journal of Nursing Administration*
Volume (Issue): 28(9)   **Year:** 1998 (September)   **Pages:** 21–27

Summary: Increasingly, hospital restructuring is viewed with skepticism because of a lack of systematic and rigorous evaluation of its impact on quality of care. This first article in a two-part series describes comprehensive evaluation of the effects of hospital restructuring on patient satisfaction, nurse satisfaction, costs of care, and clinical quality on four medical-surgical units at a large tertiary hospital. In addition, early application of the model to critical care is described. A quasi-experimental pre- and postdesign combined with concurrent control units for selected measures was the overall strategy. The authors conclude that comprehensive restructuring of hospital-based care can take place in a manner that preserves multiple dimensions of quality while decreasing costs. This only can be ascertained, however, through rigorous and systematic measurement and evaluation. Part 2 will detail application and evaluation of the restructuring model in the critical care environment.

Author(s): Bryan, Y. E., Hitchings, K. S., Fuss, M. A., Fox, M. A., Kinneman, M. T., & Young, M. J.
Article Title: Measuring and evaluating hospital restructuring efforts: Eighteen-month follow-up and extension to critical care, part 2
Journal Title: *Journal of Nursing Administration*
Volume (Issue): 28(10)   **Year:** 1998 (October)   **Pages:** 13–19

Summary: In this article, the second in a two-part series, the authors describe restructuring efforts, inclusive of their measurement and evaluation strategies, within four critical care units at an acute care, tertiary institution. Special emphasis is placed on the process, the authors' observations, and lessons learned to date. Part 1 (September 1998) presented evaluation data of the effects of hospital restructuring on patient and nurse satisfaction, costs of care, and clinical quality in four medical-surgical units.

Author(s): Cady, N., Mattes, M., & Burton, S.
Article Title: Reducing intensive care unit length of stay: A stepdown unit for first-day heart surgery patients
Journal Title: *Journal of Nursing Administration*
Volume (Issue): 25(12) **Year:** 1995 (December) **Pages:** 29–35

Summary: This article described a team approach used to design, implement, and evaluate an alternative care delivery approach at the University of Missouri Hospitals and clinics: A stepdown unit (SDU) for care of patients 24 to 36 hours after cardiothoracic surgery. Positive financial impact was reported and during the first year of the SDU, there were no negative outcomes for patients, and no patients returned to the ICU after transfer to the SDU. Implementation of this care delivery approach reportedly resulted in enhanced satisfaction of patients and families, and expectations of health care team members was reportedly exceeded expectations.

Author(s): Chang, B. L., Rubenstein, L. V., Keeler, E. B., Miura, L. N., & Kahn, K. L.
Article Title: The validity of a nursing assessment and monitoring of signs and symptoms scale in ICU and non-ICU patients
Journal Title: *American Journal of Critical Care*
Volume (Issue): 5(4) **Year:** 1996 (July) **Pages:** 298–303

Summary: This study examined the validity of medical record–based nursing assessment and monitoring of signs and symptoms (nursing surveillance) in predicting patients who were admitted to ICUs and those admitted to non-ICUs. The association of this assessment and monitoring with differences in an intermediate patient outcome, instability at discharge, was also explored. Patients admitted to either setting with a diagnosis of acute MI, cerebrovascular accident, CHF, or pneumonia were included in the study. Data from the medical records of 11,246 patients (52% female, 48% male) with a mean age of 76.4 years were used in the present study. ICU patients ($n = 3969$) were found to have a longer length of stay and to be sicker on admission than non-ICU patients ($n = 7277$). Overall, patients in the ICU received significantly higher nursing assessment and monitoring of signs and symptoms scores than non-ICU patients. Nursing assessment and monitoring of signs and symptoms scores were lower for patients discharged with greater instability for three of the four diseases (cerebrovascular accidents, CHF, and pneumonia).

Author(s): Effken, J. A., & Stetler, C. B.
Article Title: Impact of organizational redesign
Journal Title: *Journal of Nursing Administration*
Volume (Issue): 27(7/8) **Year:** 1997 (July/August) **Pages:** 23–32

Summary: This article describes a program evaluation approach used to assess and enhance large-scale organizational change in an acute care medical center,

Hartford Hospital. A variety of tools such as interviews, surveys, and various quality and cost measures were used to evaluate the integrity of innovations and to measure intermediate and end outcomes. Based on the accumulated "preponderance of evidence," it was concluded that the patient-centered redesign had made significant progress in creating an innovative, patient-centered, hospital-wide delivery system within the organization that was continuously improving quality and using resources cost effectively.

Author(s): Fuss, M. A., Bryan, Y. E., Hitchings, K. S., Fox, M. A., Kinneman, M. T., Skumanich, S., & Young, M. J.
Article Title: Measuring critical care redesign: Impact on satisfaction and quality
Journal Title: *Nursing Administration Quarterly*
Volume (Issue): 23(1) **Year:** 1998 (Fall) **Pages:** 1–14

Summary: This report describes restructuring on four critical care units at an acute, tertiary care hospital in southeast Pennsylvania. Utilizing a Patient Centered Care conceptual framework that had been successfully applied in the medical-surgical areas, restructuring involved three main areas: revamping of work processes, inclusive of redesigned staff roles; environmental and facility changes; and enhancement of telecommunication and information systems. Preliminary analyses 6 months after redesign revealed improvements and maintenance in four outcomes areas—satisfaction, quality and efficiency, and costs of care.

Author(s): Litherland, K.
Article Title: Lessons learned while implementing service quality improvement
Journal Title: *Journal for Healthcare Quality*
Volume (Issue): 17(5) **Year:** 1995 (September/October) **Pages:** 14–17

Summary: The successful implementation of quality improvement in an organization requires the organizations' executives to visibly and consistently demonstrate an understanding of and commitment to quality improvement principles. One means of developing this understanding is to give executives firsthand experience with quality improvement tools and skills. This article details the lessons learned by personnel at a large medical center during the implementation of quality improvement initiatives and highlights some aspects of the role hospital executives must play in achieving quality improvement. Whatever approach an organization chooses for the implementation of quality improvement , the exercise of discipline to do what is right inevitably will lead to the improvement of quality.

Author(s): Marino, B. L., & Ganser, C. C.
Article Title: Sensitivity of patient report of care to organizational change
Journal Title: *Journal of Nursing Administration*
Volume (Issue): 27(4) **Year:** 1997 (April) **Pages:** 32–36

Summary: The purpose of this longitudinal study was to analyze trends in patient/parent report of care over a 5-year period of major system changes in a pediatric teaching hospital to determine the degree of sensitivity of this measure to changes in nursing care. The Clinical Consumer Survey was administered by telephone to parents ($n = 3622$) of children (less than 18 years of age) within 3 weeks after discharge. There were no statistically or clinically significant differences in parent report of nursing care, evaluation of nursing care, or evaluation of length of stay. The authors concluded that patient report of care should not be the sole measure of the effect of restructuring on patients.

Author(s): Mitchell, P. H., Shannon, S. E., Cain, K. C., & Hegyvary, S.
Article Title: Critical care outcomes: Linking structures, processes, and organizational and clinical outcomes
Journal Title: *American Journal of Critical Care*
Volume (Issue): 5(5)   **Year:** 1996 (September)   **Pages:** 353–365

Summary: Quality-of-care patient and organizational outcomes were evaluated in 25 critical care units to test the hypothesis that a discretionary pattern of organizational structure and process factors is predictive of critical care unit performance, that is, desirable patient and organizational outcomes. A single value representing each critical care unit's Euclidian distance from a theoretically ideal pattern of discretionary function was determined and correlated with unit-level measures of outcomes (standardized mortality ratio, severity-adjusted length of stay, patient satisfaction, quality of nursing care, and nursing retention). Distance from the ideal-type discretionary pattern predicted organizational but not clinical outcomes. Units closer to the ideal-type pattern had higher RN retention, and were viewed as better places to work, with higher-quality care by both nurses and physicians. Objectively measured quality of care, patient satisfaction, severity-adjusted mortality, and length of stay were not consistently related to better-structured units. With experienced critical care practitioners, unit-level structure and process factors were better predictors of organizational outcomes than of clinical outcomes.

Author(s): Urden, L. D.
Article Title: Development of a nurse executive decision support database: A model for outcomes evaluation
Journal Title: *Journal of Nursing Administration*
Volume (Issue): 26(10)   **Year:** 1996 (October) **Pages:** 15–20

Summary: It is increasingly more important that nurse executives systematically evaluate innovations and changes in nursing practice and management. To plan effectively, data elements that are most appropriate for decision making must be identified and strategies for data collection and analysis must be formulated. The author describes a model in which an identifiable group of clinical, fiscal, quality, productivity, and care provider variables serve as data for baseline and later comparative evaluations.

Infection Control (N = 7)

Author(s): Brooks, K., Whitten, S., & Quigley, D.
Article Title: Reducing the incidence of ventilator-related pneumonia
Journal Title: *Journal for Healthcare Quality*
Volume (Issue): 20(1)   **Year:** 1998   **Pages:** 14–19

Summary: Ventilator-related pneumonia is costly not only in terms of treatment, equipment, and length of stay but also in terms of patient morbidity and mortality. From October 1995 through March 1996 an increase in ventilator-related pneumonia cases, of which 83% were caused by methicillin-resistant *Staphylococcus aureus* (MRSA), was noted at a Veterans Affairs medical center. A multidisciplinary team based on the TQI model and using TQI tools, methodology, and principles of problem solving was subsequently formed to look into ventilator-related pneumonia. The team's data collection and analysis efforts identified numerous opportunities for improvement. The primary outcome has been a decrease in the incidence of ventilator-related pneumonia that has resulted in substantial cost savings.

Author(s): Herchline, T., & Gros S.
Article Title: Implementation of consensus guidelines for the follow-up of positive blood cultures
Journal Title: *Infection Control & Hospital Epidemiology*
Volume (Issue): 18(1)   **Year:** 1997 (January)   **Pages:** 38–41

Summary: This prospective epidemiologic study assessed the effect and use of resources associated with implementation of a program for the systematic follow-up of positive blood cultures (BCs). There were 3121 BCs drawn, of which 199 (6.4%) were positive from 145 episodes. Sixty-three episodes involved probable contaminants, and 82 episodes were considered true bacteremias. Six patients with true bacteremia died, two were transferred, and three were discharged within 24 hours of drawing the positive BC. Of the remaining 71 true bacteremias, 9 patients were on inadequate empiric therapy, as judged by the final organism susceptibilities. Changes in empiric therapy were recommended for five of the nine episodes and were implemented by the primary physicians in each case. Each of the changes resulted in improved coverage. This program has improved the quality of care at the cost of 1 additional hour of consultant time per week.

Author(s): Mabon, B. L., Ciardi, B., Nouri, K., & Ruben, F. L.
Article Title: Concise communications. Skin testing for tuberculosis in university teaching hospitals—Is there a problem?
Journal Title: *Infection Control & Hospital Epidemiology*
Volume (Issue): 18(4)   **Year:** 1997 (April)   **Pages:** 247-249

Summary: This article describes four annual audits of tuberculin tests performed on hospitalized patients at a university teaching hospital complex. Each audit assessed if tests were performed and read correctly. House staff performed skin testing in years 1 to 3. Despite interventions of teaching and then of written instructions on skin testing, performance was poor. When testing was turned over in year 4 to trained infection control practitioners, performance approached 100%. The authors concluded that university teaching hospitals should assess skin-testing performance.

Author(s): Murphy, M., Noetscher, C., & Lagoe, R.
Article Title: A multihospital effort to reduce inpatient lengths of stay for pneumonia
Journal Title: *Journal of Nursing Care Quality*
Volume (Issue): 13(5) **Year:** 1999 (June) **Pages:** 11–23

Summary: Three large hospitals in the metropolitan area of Syracuse, New York, implemented a cooperative project to reduce hospital stays and resource utilization without adversely affecting patient outcomes for community-acquired pneumonia. The project occurred under the leadership of nurse case managers and nurse managers. It was supported by active physician involvement. The project was implemented over a 3-year period. It resulted in reductions of hospital stays through the standardization of patient care for pneumonia throughout the community.

Author(s): Nicotra, D., & Ulrich, C.
Article Title: Process improvement plan for the reduction of nosocomial pneumonia in patients on ventilators
Journal Title: *Journal of Nursing Care Quality*
Volume (Issue): 10(4) **Year:** 1996 (July) **Pages:** 18–23

Summary: In one hospital, after the discovery of a ventilator-associated nosocomial infection rate that was higher than the national standard, a multidisciplinary team was formed. The team followed the FOCUS-PDCA model of quality improvement to identify methods to improve the nosocomial pneumonia infection rate for mechanically ventilated patients. Three areas of potential improvement were identified: trial of a closed suction system, policies and procedures for cleaning of ventilators, and staff education. Additionally, a research project was conducted to identify predictors of ventilator-associated nosocomial pneumonia. These projects resulted in a reduction of the ventilator-associated nosocomial pneumonia infection rate to 8.3/1000 ventilator days and a cost savings of more than $580,000.

Author(s): Phillips, K. F., & Crain, H. C.
Article Title: Effectiveness of a pneumonia clinical pathway: Quality and financial outcomes
Journal Title: *Outcomes Management for Nursing Practice*
Volume (Issue): 2(1) **Year:** 1998 (January–March) **Pages:** 16–23

Summary: In today's health care environment, it is imperative to evaluate planned changes within a health care system. This article reports the outcomes of a study on the effectiveness of a pneumonia clinical pathway. Important elements of effectiveness studies are discussed and used in presenting study findings. These findings are a preliminary demonstration that clinical pathways can improve patient and process outcomes. Their relation to financial outcomes is less clear.

Author(s): Simonds, D. N., Horan, T. C., Kelley, R., & Jarvis, W. R.
Article Title: Detecting pediatric nosocomial infections: How do infection control and quality assurance personnel compare?
Journal Title: *American Journal of Infection Control*
Volume (Issue): 25(3)   **Year:** 1997 (June)   **Pages:** 202–208

Summary: This study was designed to compare how well infection control (IC) and quality assurance (QA) personnel in a specialty setting identify the presence, type (nosocomial or community-acquired), and (if nosocomial) site of infection. In 1994, a survey that included 21 pediatric case histories was mailed to IC and QA personnel in pediatric settings in the United States. From the case histories presented, the respondents were asked to determine whether an infection was present and, if so, whether it was nosocomial or community-acquired. If the infection was nosocomial, the respondent was asked to determine the site of the infection (e.g., urinary tract, blood stream). One hundred thirty-one respondents (45.3%) completed 212 surveys. IC and QA personnel were similar in ability to identify community-acquired infection. IC personnel were significantly more likely than QA personnel to accurately identify the specific sites of infection. Overall, IC personnel were more accurate than QA personnel in determining whether a nosocomial infection was present and in correctly determining most sites of infection. Both IC and QA personnel had difficulty identifying venous infection and respiratory tract infection with secondary bloodstream infection. In addition, QA personnel did not perform overall as well as IC personnel in identifying nosocomial infections and their sites; this finding suggests the need for QA personnel to be provided specific training on detection of nosocomial infections and validation of their ability to do so.

Specific Clinical Issues Related to Patient Populations (N = 28)

Author(s): Anderson, M. A., & Helms, L. B.
Article Title: Extended care referral after hospital discharge
Journal Title: *Research in Nursing & Health*
Volume (Issue): 21(5) **Year:** 1998 (October) **Pages:** 385–394

Summary: The purpose of this nonexperimental, retrospective, descriptive study was to describe patient-related information and selected organizational and medical factors in referrals of elderly patients following discharge by acute care hospitals to extended care facilities (ECFs). Four hundred fifty-five closed records of referral to ECFs by acute care hospitals were analyzed. The Referral Data Inventory (RDI) measured the amount and type of information an ECF receives upon referral of an elderly patient from a hospital. The total amount of data transferred in the ECF referral of elderly patients upon discharge from an acute care hospital was reflected in a score on the RDI between 0 and 40, with higher scores indicating larger amounts of data sent. Hospitals transferred over three-fourths of the literature-recommended amount of patient care data. Referrals contained primarily background and medical, followed by nursing care and psychosocial data. Specialty units in hospitals transferred more content-rich patient referrals than general medical-surgical units. Findings from this study suggest the relationship of structural and economic factors and the potential role of technology in interorganizational communication between health care providers concerning patients referred for continuing care.

Author(s): Blewitt, D. K., & Jones, K. R.
Article Title: Using elements of the nursing minimum data set for determining outcomes
Journal Title: *Journal of Nursing Administration*
Volume (Issue): 26(6) **Year:** 1996 (June) **Pages:** 48–56

Summary: This exploratory-descriptive pilot study explored the utilization of elements of the Nursing Minimum Data Set (NMDS) in a sample of patients undergoing parathyroidectomy in a major academic medical center setting. Data collected from patients enrolled in larger study being conducted on surgical outcomes were used and sources of data included patients ($n = 20$), nurses ($n = 10$), and medical record review. Comparison between expected outcomes identified by nurses and patients demonstrated incongruence between nurse and patient expectations for the outcomes of surgery. Inconsistent use and documentation of the critical data elements and nursing diagnoses, goals, and associated interventions made it impossible to establish a clear link between nursing activities and patient outcomes in this study. Results support the importance of nursing management's role in creating reliable systems that capture the critical elements of care delivery.

Author(s): Bromenshenkel, J., Newcomb, M., & Thompson, J.
Article Title: Continuous quality improvement efforts decrease postoperative ileus rates
Journal Title: *Journal for Healthcare Quality*
Volume (Issue): 22(2)   **Year:** 2000 (March/April)   **Pages:** 4-7

Summary: This study examined the impact of a CQI program on the occurrence of postoperative ileus in selected patients in a 98-bed acute care facility located in the northeastern United States. Upon evaluation of the program, 6 months following implementation overall rates were found to be lower in patients having five selected surgical procedures. Overall ileus rates were reported to be 1.9% in 1997, down from 4.8% in 1995.

Author(s): Bultema, J. K., Mailliard, L., Getzfrid, M. K., Lerner, R. D., & Colone, M.
Article Title: Geriatric patients with depression: Improving outcomes using a multidisciplinary clinical path model
Journal Title: *Journal of Nursing Administration*
Volume (Issue): 26(1)   **Year:** 1996 (January)   **Pages:** 31–38

Summary: This article describes the development and implementation of a psychiatric clinical pathway for geriatric patients with depression, and identified common multidisciplinary interventions and a pattern of outcomes after treatment for these patients in Northwestern Memorial Hospital, an urban academic medical center in the Midwest. A pilot study, comparing a random sample of 12 patients assigned to the pathway with 12 patients treated before pathway implementation, identified significant quality improvements. Decreased cost per case and length of stay were positive fiscal outcomes reported.

Author(s): Burden, B., & Taft, E.
Article Title: A data-driven approach to improving clinical outcomes in cardiac care
Journal Title: *Journal for Healthcare Quality*
Volume (Issue): 21(2)   **Year:** 1999   **Pages:** 32–36

Summary: This study of clinical outcomes used clinical outcomes of mortality, emergent or urgent return of cardiac surgery patient to the operating room (OR), and development of cardiac surgery complications such as cerebral vascular accident as indicators of quality. Data were tracked using facility and national clinical cardiac databases, with quarterly facility and individual practitioner reports provided. Case review was also used to monitor indicators. Focused continuing medical education was provided, which focused on problems identified. Decreases were reported in mortality rates following CABG and decreases in other complication rates such as emergent return to the OR, postoperative bleeding, and emergent CABG after percutaneous transluminal coronary angioplasty (PTCA). The author suggests that changes were related to increased attention to processes of care and heightened physician awareness of data tracking and scrutiny.

Author(s): Card, S. J., Herrling, P. J., Matthews, J. L., Rossi, M. L., Spencer, E. S., & Lagoe, R.
Article Title: Impact of clinical pathways for total hip replacement: A community-based analysis
Journal Title: *Journal of Nursing Care Quality*
Volume (Issue): 13(2)   **Year:** 1998 (December)   **Pages:** 67–76

Summary: The implementation of clinical pathways for total hip replacement was carried out by five hospitals in the metropolitan area of Syracuse, New York. This process occurred under the leadership of clinical nurse specialists and nurse managers. It was supported by preadmission patient education programs and active physician involvement. The participating hospitals shared utilization QA data and benchmarked with respect to the experience of Sacramento, California, and each others' progress. The effort produced substantial reductions in hospital stays without adverse impacts on quality of care.

Author(s): Cardozo, L., & Aherns, S.
Article Title: Assessing the efficacy of a clinical pathway in the management of older patients hospitalized with congestive heart failure
Journal Title: *Journal for Healthcare Quality*
Volume (Issue): 21(3)   **Year:** 1999   **Pages:** 12–17

Summary: This article compares outcomes in a group of older hospitalized patients managed on a CHF pathway with those of a historical cohort managed in the traditional manner. The patients on the pathway had significant reductions in length of stay and cost of care as well as more effective delivery of processes of care. Mortality rates were unchanged, at 3.5%. However, readmission rates showed a significant increase, from 9.25 to 13.5%, for patients on the pathway.

Author(s): Crawley, W. D.
Article Title: Case management: Improving outcomes of care for ischemic stroke patients
Journal Title: *MEDSURG Nursing*
Volume (Issue): 5(4)   **Year:** 1996 (August)   **Pages:** 239–244

Summary: Stroke is a leading cause of death and disability in the United States. Health care reform and escalating health care costs have caused both consumers and health care providers to become more concerned regarding health care provision for stroke patients. A case management practice model used in a 540-bed teaching hospital resulted in improved outcomes for ischemic stroke patients in the areas of (a) functional ability, (b) appointment compliance, (c) length of stay, and (d) cost.

Author(s): Cushing, K. A., & Stratta, R. J.
Article Title: Design, development, and implementation of a critical pathway in simultaneous pancreas-kidney transplant recipients
Journal Title: *Journal of Transplant Coordination*
Volume (Issue): 7(4)   **Year:** 1997 (December)   **Pages:** 164–172

Summary: The purpose of this study was to assess the effect of implementation of a critical pathway after simultaneous pancreas-kidney transplantation on length of stay and hospital charges. Two well-matched groups were compared: 10 patients who received transplants in 1991 (before implementation of the critical pathway) and 10 patients who received transplants in 1995 (after implementation). For the initial transplant hospitalization, the critical pathway was associated with significant reductions in length of stay, total number of laboratory tests, clinical laboratory charges, and total inpatient charges (with organ acquisition charges excluded). Despite the rising costs of medical care, the critical pathway designed and implemented for simultaneous pancreas-kidney transplantation has stabilized hospital charges by decreasing length of stay and the number of clinical laboratory tests.

Author(s): Griffin, H., Davis, L., Gant, E., Savona, M., Shaw, L., Strickland, J., Wood, C., & Wagner, G.
Article Title: A community hospital's effort to expedite treatment for patients with chest pain
Journal Title: *Heart & Lung: Journal of Acute & Critical Care*
Volume (Issue): 28(6)   **Year:** 1999 (November–December)   **Pages:** 402–408

Summary: The purpose of this descriptive study was to determine treatment times at a community hospital that does not receive prehospital electrocardiogram (ECG) transmission and to determine the effect of time to first hospital ECG on overall door-to-drug time. One hundred four patients with a final diagnosis of acute MI were included in this 16-month study. A median door-to-ECG time of 5 minutes was within the American College of Cardiology/American Heart Association recommendation of 10 minutes. Shorter treatment times to obtain the first ECG and initiate thrombolytic therapy were associated with younger patients and those arriving by ambulance. Although efficiency in obtaining a first hospital ECG on patients with suspected acute MIs was achieved, this did not result in low door-to-drug times. Further streamlining of protocol and the exploration of prehospital initiatives may result in a significant reduction in door-to-drug times.

Author(s): Hall, G. R., Karstens, M., Rakel, B., Swanson, E., & Davidson, A.
Article Title: Managing constipation using a research-based protocol
Journal Title: *MEDSURG Nursing*
Volume (Issue): 4(1)   **Year:** 1995 (February)   **Pages:** 11–20

Summary: As part of a quality improvement initiative, a research-based interdisciplinary protocol was developed to prevent constipation in hospitalized immobile vascular surgery patients. Using a combination of dietary fiber, increased fluid, and hygiene measures over a 3-year period, incidence of constipation was reduced from 59% to about 9%. The incidence of impaction was eliminated and requests for laxatives and enemas were reduced from 59% to about 8%.

Author(s): Hamilton, L., & Lyon, P. S.
Article Title: A nursing-driven program to preserve and restore functional ability in hospitalized elderly patients
Journal Title: *Journal of Nursing Administration*
Volume (Issue): 25(4)   **Year:** 1995 (April)   **Pages:** 30–37

Summary: This study used a quasi-experimental, one-group pre-/posttest design to test the effectiveness of institutionally developed, multidisciplinary, geriatric acute care modules for assessment and rehabilitation. Three resource manuals were developed for the modules: (1) *Urinary Continence in the Elderly*, (2) *Improving Functional Mobility in the Elderly: A Nursing Program, and* (3) *The Geriatric Module Manual* (policies and procedures). The dependent variable was functional status, as measured by the Modified Barthel Index. Although many of the subjects ($N = 74$) had some degree of cognitive impairment, enhanced nursing enabled them to make significant gains in their functional abilities.

Author(s): Heckman, M., Ajdari, S. Y., Esquivel, M., Chernof, B., Tamm, N., Landowski, L., & Guterman, J. J.
Article Title: Quality improvement principles in practice: The reduction of umbilical cord blood errors in the labor and delivery suite
Journal Title: *Journal of Nursing Care Quality*
Volume (Issue): 12(3)   **Year:** 1998 (February)   **Pages:** 47–54

Summary: Mislabeled umbilical cord blood specimens were identified as an important and difficult problem to solve. Quality improvement principles were employed after education-based interventions failed to achieve measurable improvement. A small interdisciplinary working group of key stakeholders investigated, designed, and evaluated interventions for a solution. This article describes a system-based change where substantial qualitative and quantitative improvements were measured. The success of the change is attributed to the involvement and commitment by key stakeholders and use of systems re-engineering principles.

Author(s): Homes, L. M., & Hollabaugh, S. K.
Article Title: Using the continuous quality improvement process to improve the care of patients after angioplasty
Journal Title: *Critical Care Nurse*
Volume (Issue): 17(6)   **Year:** 1997 (December)   **Pages:** 56–60, 62–65

Summary: Although care and removal of arterial sheaths are becoming routine practice in most coronary care units and some telemetry units, no standard of care exists for when these sheaths should be removed in relation to the reversal of systemic anticoagulation. In this article, optimal times are defined for removal of arteriovenous sheaths after PTCA once systematic administration of heparin has been discontinued. The process used to develop this standard of care and the outcomes achieved are also described.

Author(s): Maxey, C.

Article Title: A case map reduces time to administration of thrombolytic therapy in patients experiencing an acute myocardial infarction

Journal Title: *Nursing Case Management*

Volume (Issue): 2(5) **Year:** 1997 (September–October) **Pages:** 229–237

Summary: To monitor quality in lytic therapy administration, one hospital began to participate in the National Registry for Myocardial Infarction (NRMI) in January, 1995. The first quarter of data revealed a median door-to-drug time (time from arrival at hospital to administration of drug) of 67 minutes. As a quality improvement project, a research experiment was conducted to assess the effect of a case map, also referred to as a clinical pathway, on time to administration of thrombolytic therapy. The researcher developed a case map designed to increase efficiency in delivery of thrombolytic agents. The research was conducted over an 18-month period from July 1995 to December 1996. Median time to administration of thrombolytic therapy was reduced from 64 to 25 minutes as a result of case map use ($p = .028$).

Author(s): Meier, P. P., Engstrom, J. L., Fleming, B. A., Streeter, P. L., & Lawrence, P. B.

Article Title: Estimating milk intake of hospitalized preterm infants who breastfeed

Journal Title: *Journal of Human Lactation*

Volume (Issue): 12(1) **Year:** 1996 **Pages:** 21–26

Summary: This study describes the accuracy of clinical indices to estimate the milk intake of breastfed preterm infants. Twenty-nine mother–infant pairs were studied for a total of 39 breastfeeding sessions. Clinical indices did not provide an accurate estimate of milk intake ($r = .48$). The mean absolute difference between the test weights and clinical estimates was 5.79 ml, with a maximal difference of 20 ml. These differences were random in that clinical indices did not consistently over- or underestimate milk intake. None of 17 clinical indices of milk intake significantly lowered the magnitude of error in the clinical estimate. These data suggest that clinical indices cannot serve as a replacement for test weighing of preterm infants when an accurate estimate of milk intake is necessary.

Author(s): Oetker, D., & Cole, C.

Article Title: Improving the outcome of emergency department patients with a chief complaint of chest pain

Journal Title: *Journal of Nursing Care Quality*

Volume (Issue): 10(2) **Year:** 1996 (January) **Pages:** 58–74

Summary: Preliminary data developed by the Health Care Financing Administration (HCFA) indicate that 50% of Medicare heart attack patients arriving in ED who are candidates for thrombolytic therapy do not receive it within the time period specified by the American College of Cardiology. Indicators developed for QA monitoring and evaluation of a hospital ED prompted closer review of some cases. It was determined that a critical outcomes team using the principles of TQM and the FOCUS-PDCA models should be empowered to deal with these issues. Through this process, the need for the development of a chest pain center at the hospital was identified and supported.

Author(s): Painter, L. M., Dudjak, L. A., Breiner, K., & Langford A.
Article Title: Abdominal aortic aneurysm pathway: Outcome analysis
Journal Title: *Journal of Vascular Nursing*
Volume (Issue): 13(4)   **Year:** 1995   **Pages:** 101–105

Summary: The purpose of this study was to describe a process for analysis of clinical and fiscal outcomes of a clinical pathway initiated at an academic medical center for elective abdominal aortic aneurysm repair. Patients were monitored throughout their pre- and postoperative course to identify and trend variances, assess opportunities for improved resource use, and determine patient/family satisfaction. Results of a sample of 42 patients revealed a reduction in gross charges by 33% per case in comparison to the baseline data obtained before pathway implementation. Clinical outcomes and related nursing implications were discussed, including preoperative management, a streamlined same-day admission process, and factors associated with prolonged stay in the ICU.

Author(s): Philbin, E. F., Rogers, V. A., Sheesley, K. A., Lynch, L. J., Andreou, C., & Rocco, T.A. Jr.
Article Title: The relationship between hospital length of stay and rate of death in heart failure
Journal Title: *Heart & Lung: Journal of Acute & Critical Care*
Volume (Issue): 26(3)   **Year:** 1997 (May–June)   **Pages:** 177–186

Summary: A retrospective, observational study examined the relationship between length of stay (LOS) and the rate of death among patients hospitalized with CHF. Significant variability in mean total LOS, mean acute LOS, and death rates was noted among the centers. Minimal variation in mean expected LOS and mean severity score was observed. Mean total LOS and acute LOS were not related significantly to death rate for the 15 centers. When the hospitals were separated into tertiles based on rank order of total LOS and acute LOS, no differences among the subgroups were noted in the number of cases per hospital, deaths per hospital, death rates, expected LOS, or severity scores. Interhospital variation in total LOS was partially explained by the care of patients who did not require acute hospitalization. Significant interhospital variation exists in LOS and death rates for patients admitted with CHF; these two measures are not related. This variability in outcome cannot be explained by severity of illness case-mix alone; significant variation in the processes and effectiveness of patient care may exist.

Author(s): Philbin, E. F., Lynch, L. J., Rocco, T. A., Lindenmuth, N. W., Ulrich, K., McCall, M., Jenkins, P., & Roerden, J. B.
Article Title: Does QI work? The Management to Improve Survival in Congestive Heart Failure (MISCHF) study
Journal Title: *Journal on Quality Improvement*
Volume (Issue): 22(11)   **Year:** 1996   **Pages:** 721–733

Summary: As a randomized, controlled clinical trial, this study was designed to measure the efficacy of a program on changing clinical practice patterns; as a clinical quality improvement initiative, the study was designed to improve patient outcomes.

Author(s): Rantz, M., Davis, N. K., & Tapp, R. A.
Article Title: Assessing elderly acute care services: Improving quality amid chaos
Journal Title: *Journal of Nursing Care Quality*
Volume (Issue): 9(3)   **Year:** 1995   **Pages:** 1–9

Summary: Elderly service delivery within the medical-surgical division of a large Midwestern tertiary care center was assessed to explore how to better meet the special needs and address the complex situation s that older adults present. Participant observation and unstructured interviews were used to collect data in four medical-surgical units and a medical-surgical ICU. The following categories emerged from the qualitative data analysis: problems related to the care of older adults, causes of confusion, effective and potentially effective interventions for older patients, and staff educational needs.

Author(s): Riegel, B., Gates, D. M., Gocka, I., Medina, L., Odell, C., Rich, M., & Finken, J. S.
Article Title: Effectiveness of a program of early hospital discharge of cardiac surgery patients [corrected] [published erratum appears in *J Cardiovasc Nurs* 1997 Apr; 11(3): viii].
Journal Title: *Journal of Cardiovascular Nursing*
Volume (Issue): 11(1)   **Year:** 1996 (October)   **Pages:** 63–75

Summary: Managed care was the impetus for a program designed to move adult patients from acute care to the lowest level of appropriate services after cardiac surgery. Clinical pathways and a home care cardiac specialty team were the major components of the Early Discharge Program. A convenience sample of 119 pretest patients was compared with 101 posttest patients 3 months after program implementation. Hospital length of stay decreased only 0.34 days on average, but inpatient direct variable costs decreased by an average of $1,790 per patient. Based on the 101 patients in the posttest group, $180,790 in direct variable hospital costs were saved. The largest decrease in resource use was in those patients who were discharged to home care. Complications and home caregiver burden after discharge were no higher for patients discharged early. Early discharge of cardiac surgery patients appears to be safe and cost effective.

Author(s): Roman, S., Linekin, P., & Stagnaro-Green, A.
Article Title: An inpatient diabetes QI program
Journal Title: *The Joint Commission Journal on Quality Improvement*
Volume (Issue): 21(12)   **Year:** 1995   **Pages:** 693–699

Summary: The goal of this study was to establish a CQI program for diabetes to identify patterns in the problems of care encountered by hospitalized patients with diabetes and improve the in-hospital process of diabetes care delivery. Documentation of nursing unit-based capillary blood glucose monitoring

(CBGM) and insulin infusion monitoring improved significantly over time. The medical management of hypoglycemia, hyperglycemia, and diabetic ketoacidosis (DKA) improved over the 3-year period. Efforts to standardize specific clinical and documentation processes had a positive impact on the care of hospitalized patients with diabetes and resulted in an institutional effort to improve inpatient diabetes care with a CQI team.

Author(s): Rumble, S. J., Jernigan, M. H., & Rudisill, P. T.
Article Title: Determining the effectiveness of critical pathways for coronary bypass graft patients: Retrospective comparison of readmission rates
Journal Title: *Journal of Nursing Care Quality*
Volume (Issue): 11(2)   **Year:** 1996 (December)   **Pages:** 34–40

Summary: The article describes a study performed to determine whether the use of the critical path tool made a difference in the readmission rates of patients after CABG surgery compared with CABG patients cared for without the critical path tool. The sample for this retrospective study consisted of 780 specific patient medical records from the medical record department. Examination of these data revealed no statistically significant difference in readmission for CABG patients cared for with critical paths and those cared for without critical paths. A comparison of hospital length of stay and surgical length of stay between the two groups, however, revealed statistically significant differences between the two groups. The critical path group had a significant decrease in hospital and surgical length of stay.

Author(s): Shedd, P. P., Kobokovich, L. J., & Slattery, J. S.
Article Title: Confused patients in the acute care setting: Prevalence, interventions, and outcomes
Journal Title: *Journal of Gerontological Nursing*
Volume (Issue): 21(4)   **Year:** 1995 (April)   **Pages:** 5–12

Summary: A descriptive design was used to measure nurses' assessment of the prevalence of patients who are confused, the interventions used, and these patients' outcomes on three nursing units in an acute care setting. Confused patients had less favorable outcomes at discharge than did the group of non-confused patients. Of the three interventions that were monitored, confused patients were more likely to have either restraints or medications than to have a sitter (a sitter is a paid staff member or a family member who monitored the patient directly).

Author(s): Wammack, L., & Mabrey, J. D.
Article Title: Outcomes assessment of total hip and total knee arthroplasty: Critical pathways, variance analysis, and continuous quality improvement
Journal Title: *Clinical Nurse Specialist*
Volume (Issue): 12(3)   **Year:** 1998 (May)   **Pages:** 122–131

Summary: Using critical pathways, with variance analysis and CQI techniques to refine the pathways, the efficiency of total hip and total knee surgeries in one academic health center was maximized. Using a retrospective cohort study design, complications, readmissions, morbidity/mortality, and function scores were examined in two groups of patients attended by the same surgeon for the year before and the year after the implementation of an outcomes management program. The length of stay was reduced by 57% for knee patients and 46% for hip patients. Hospital costs were reduced 11% for all knees and 38% for hips. Complications were also significantly reduced. There was no statistically significant difference between pre- and postoperative knee or hip outcome scores. The program resulted in significant savings without adversely affecting overall outcome.

Author(s): Whitcomb, R., & Aleman, D.
Article Title: Achieving excellence in thrombolytic therapy
Journal Title: *Journal for Healthcare Quality*
Volume (Issue): 17(3)   **Year:** 1995 (May/June)   **Pages:** 23–25, 38

Summary: Thrombolytic therapy for patients with acute MI can present challenges to ED and critical care nursing staff. The areas of concomitant medications, screening checklists, associated laboratory studies, and overall time to treatment presented opportunities for improvement at a Florida hospital. The clinical process and the existing quality improvement activities were reviewed by a multidisciplinary CQI team. The outcomes of the CQI process were extremely favorable; 100% compliance was achieved in all aspects of care for patients with acute MI.

Author(s): York, R., Brown, L. P., Samuels, P., Finkler, S. A., Jacobsen, B., Persely, C. A., Swank, A., & Robbins, D.
Article Title: A randomized trial of early discharge and nurse specialist transitional follow-up care of high-risk childbearing women
Journal Title: *Nursing Research*
Volume (Issue): 46(5)   **Year:** 1997 (September-October)   **Pages:** 254–261

Summary: In a randomized clinical trial, quality of health care as reflected in patient outcomes and cost of health care was compared between two groups of high-risk childbearing women: women diagnosed with diabetes or hypertension in pregnancy. The control group ($n = 52$) was discharged routinely from the hospital. The intervention group ($n = 44$) was discharged early using a model of clinical nurse specialist transitional follow-up care. During pregnancy, the intervention group had significantly fewer rehospitalizations than the control group. For infants of diabetic women enrolled in the study during their pregnancy, low birth weight (≤ 2500 g) was three times more prevalent in the control group (29%) than in the intervention group (8.3%). The postpartum hospital charges for the intervention group were also significantly lower than for the control group. The mean total hospital charges for the intervention group were 44% less than for the control group. The mean cost of the clinical specialist follow-up care was 2% of the total hospital charges for the control group. A net savings of $13,327 was realized for each mother–infant dyad discharged early from the hospital.

Clinical Issues Related to Care Processes (N = 10)

Author(s): Burris, G. W., & Jacobs, A. J.
Article Title: A continuous quality improvement process to increase organ and tissue donation
Journal Title: *Journal of Transplant Coordination*
Volume (Issue): 6(2) **Year:** 1996 (June) **Pages:** 88–92

Summary: The Omnibus Budget Reconciliation Act of 1987 mandated that hospitals must identify potential organ and tissue donors, notify an organ procurement organization of the potential donor, and inform family members regarding the opportunity to donate organs and tissues. Although JCAHO requires that hospitals comply with this statute, no standard for documenting compliance exists. A CQI process was developed at one institution to define a policy, educate staff, and document and monitor compliance. The number of referrals to the organ procurement organization and the number of organ and tissue donors were found to increase. These observations suggest that implementation of a CQI process that ensures compliance with organ procurement regulations might increase the number of organ and tissue donors.

Author(s): Carveth, J. A.
Article Title: Perceived patient deviance and avoidance by nurses
Journal Title: *Nursing Research*
Volume (Issue): 44(3) **Year:** 1995 (May–June) **Pages:** 173–178

Summary: Perceived patient deviance and its relationship to avoidance behaviors of nurses was examined using a social deviance/labeling framework. Avoidance included a reduction in the number and duration of nursing contacts with patients, a reduction in the number of nurse-initiated contacts, the use of physical restraints, and failure to meet the individualized needs of patients. Fifty-two RNs on adult health units classified known patients into three study groups: ideal patient, neutral patient, and difficult (deviant) patient. Analysis of variance showed no significant differences for mean number, duration, and initiator of nurse–patient contacts. Significant differences were found in the Psychosocial Individual, Physical, and General subscales of the Slater Nursing Competencies Rating Scale and in the use of physical restraints for the three study groups. Agreement of nurses in their classification of patients occurred in 74.63% of cases. The results suggest that the label of difficult (deviant) patient is well-communicated among nurses and that it has a negative influence on the quality of care.

Author(s): Dearborn, P., De Muth, J. S., Requarth, A. B., & Ward, S. E.
Article Title: Nurse and patient satisfaction with three types of venous access devices
Journal Title: *Oncology Nursing Forum*
Volume (Issue): 24(1 Suppl) **Year:** 1997 (January–February) **Pages:** 34–40

Summary: A descriptive, correlational QA study examined patient and nurse satisfaction with three types of venous access devices (VADs)—port, Groshong

(Bard Access Systems, Salt Lake City, Utah), and Hickman (Bard Access Systems)—and to identify the problems and benefits experienced with each type of device. Consecutive patients meeting study criteria were invited to complete self-report questionnaires at the time of their clinic visits. Clinic nurses who cared for these patients also completed questionnaires. Patients' reports of benefits did not differ by device, but they reported fewer blood-drawing problems with ports than with Groshong or Hickman catheters. Patients and nurses reported infections and clots more often with Groshong catheters than with the other two devices. Patients indicated that health care workers seemed most knowledgeable about Hickman catheters. Patients with ports reported more problems with access to the device, development of hematomas, and anxiety. Nurses reported more flow rate problems with Groshong catheters than with Hickman catheters. Patients and nurses reported no flow rate problems with ports. Each device was associated with a specific problem, yet in the global satisfaction ratings, patients expressed the greatest satisfaction with Hickman catheters and ports. Nurses tended to be least satisfied with Groshong catheters. A need exists for continued patient education on VAD care to minimize complications. The selection of an appropriate VAD should be based on the patient's best interests rather than on nurses' preferences.

Author(s): Harris, J. L., & Maguire, D.
Article Title: Developing a protocol to prevent and treat pediatric central venous catheter occlusions
Journal Title: *Journal of Intravenous Nursing*
Volume (Issue): 22(4)   **Year:** 1999 (July–August)   **Pages:** 194–198

Summary: Catheter occlusions are a common occurrence in pediatric patients with central venous catheters. These occlusions are attributable to many factors, such as mechanical problems caused by catheter and patient size, clot formation caused by blood product administration and laboratory sampling, drug precipitation, and lipid residues. Because of the significant patient risk and cost involved in replacing occluded central venous catheters, a multidisciplinary team used a quality improvement approach to determine the effectiveness of urokinase in pediatric patients. Data from the project enabled development of a decision tree for urokinase use. Statistics from the pilot revealed that 85% of catheter occlusions were related to thrombotic events, and urokinase was effective in all cases. However, 15% of central line occlusions were related to medication precipitates and were not effectively cleared with urokinase. Given the evidence, urokinase is effective only on fibrin-related occlusions caused by medication precipitates.

Author(s): Hill, M. G., Fieselmann, J. F., Nobiling, H. E., O'Neill, P. S., Barry-Walker, J., Dwyer, J., & Kobler, L.
Article Title: Preventing cardiopulmonary arrest via enhanced vital signs monitoring
Journal Title: *MEDSURG Nursing*
Volume (Issue): 4(4)   **Year:** 1995   **Pages:** 289–295

Summary: A physician–nurse collaborative team developed and implemented a research-based protocol and algorithm for improving vital signs monitoring and early intervention for at-risk patients. Project evaluation showed that in general the protocol and algorithm were used appropriately and consistently and prevented negative patient outcomes.

Author(s): Jackson, G., & Andrew, J.
Article Title: Using a multidisciplinary CQI approach to reduce ER-to-floor admission time
Journal Title: *Journal for Healthcare Quality*
Volume (Issue): 18(3) **Year:** 1996 (May/June) **Pages:** 18–21

Summary: A 110-bed community hospital used a multidisciplinary continuous quality improvement process to decrease the time needed to admit a non-critical care patient to the hospital from the ED. The specific objective was to reduce the total amount of time needed for a patient who has entered the ED to be assigned to a bed on a designated medical-surgical unit, while at the same time maintaining quality of care and providing the patient with a pleasant atmosphere.

Author(s): McArthur, C. L. III, & Rooke, C. T.
Article Title: Are spinal precautions necessary in all seizure patients? . . . presented at SAEM, Toronto, May 1992
Journal Title: *American Journal of Emergency Medicine*
Volume (Issue): 13(5) **Year:** 1995 (September) **Pages:** 512–513

Summary: The purpose of this retrospective chart review study was to evaluate the necessity of spinal precautions in uncomplicated seizure patients. The population was all patients from the ED in one hospital with a primary diagnosis of seizure over a 10.5-year period. The key outcome measure was an association of spinal injuries to uncomplicated seizures. A total of 1656 cases were reviewed. No spinal injuries were found. Three nonspinal fractures were associated with seizure activity. Transportation costs increased approximately 113% and nursing costs increased approximately 57% for patients with seizure placed in spinal precautions. QA and risk management files showed no complaints or litigation secondary to missed spinal injuries. This study seriously questions routine use of spinal precautions in uncomplicated seizure cases. If spinal precautions were not used in this group, there would be significant potential cost savings without increased morbidity. A prospective study is needed to confirm these findings.

Author(s): Miller, K. D., & Deitrick, C. L.
Article Title: Experience with PICC at a University Medical Center [corrected] [published erratum appears in *J Intravenous Nurs* 1997 Jul–Aug; 20(4): 206].
Journal Title: *Journal of Intravenous Nursing*
Volume (Issue): 20(3) **Year:** 1997 (May–June) **Pages:** 141–147

Summary: This study is a retrospective evaluation of the use of the peripherally inserted central catheters inserted by a small, credentialed nursing staff to provide ongoing venous access in the general adult and pediatric patient population at the University of Rochester Medical Center in Rochester, New York. Between 1993 and 1995, 602 catheters were inserted in 775 suitable patients. Correct catheter tip placement in the superior vena cava was achieved in 95% of placements with a catheter dwell time ranging from less than 1 day to 353 days (average, 24 days). Strict adherence to obtaining and monitoring QA kept catheter complications to a minimum.

Author(s): Siminoff, L. A., Erlen, J. A., & Sereika, S.
Article Title: Do nurses avoid AIDS patients? Avoidance behaviors and the quality of care of hospitalized AIDS patients
Journal Title: *AIDS Care*
Volume (Issue): 10(2)   Year: 1998 (April)   Pages: 147–163

Summary: To examine whether patients with acquired immunodeficiency syndrome (AIDS) are stigmatized by nurses providing their care a study was conducted with 100 matched AIDS and general medical patients. Quality of care and avoidance behaviors were measured by direct, systematic observation during a concurrent 12-hour period. Stigmatizing attitudes of nurses were measured using standardized instruments of homophobia, fear of AIDS and attitudes toward illicit drug use. Nurses made more eye contact and touched AIDS patients more frequently then general medical patients, however these differences did not reach the level of statistical significance. Whether or not nurses were fearful of HIV infection, were homophobic or held negative feelings about drug use made no difference in the level of care provided to AIDS patients, but did for general medical patients. However, avoidance behaviors were associated with lower quality of care across all patients regardless of diagnosis. It was concluded that nurses' attitudes had no impact on whether or not AIDS patients were shunned by nurses. The provision of psychosocial care showed the greatest variation and seemed more sensitive to individual nurses' attitudes. The quality of care received by the overwhelming majority of patients could only be termed adequate. Nurses exhibited the greatest caution when performing procedures with patients whose HIV status was unknown.

Author(s): Wise, L. C., Mersch, J., Racioppi, J., Crosier, J., & Thompson, C.
Article Title: Evaluating the reliability and utility of cumulative intake and output
Journal Title: *Journal of Nursing Care Quality*
Volume (Issue): 14(3)   Year: 2000 (April)   Pages: 37–42

Summary: Three nurse-managers of nursing units serving diverse patient populations studied the effectiveness of continuous intake and output in estimating daily fluid balance. They examined 48-hour records of daily weight and intake and output of 73 patients and correlated the two. Their findings suggest that even when caregiver charting compliance is optimal, daily intake and output recording provides unreliable results. The authors recommend daily weights alone be adopted for all patients who are not experiencing acute renal conditions.

Work Environment (N = 8)

Author(s): Aiken, L. H., Sloane, D. M., & Sochalski, J.
Article Title: Hospital organization and outcomes
Journal Title: *Quality in Health Care*
Volume (Issue): 7(4)   **Year:** 1998 (December)   **Pages:** 222–226

Summary: This article identifies research that has been done by various investigators on hospital organization and patient outcomes, describes some of the authors recent research on that relation, and comments on where additional research is needed. A clinical environment index was used to develop three subscales measuring nurse autonomy, nurse control over the practice setting, and relations between nurses and physicians. Indicators of nurse autonomy, control over practice environment, and favorable nurse–physician relations were found to be significantly more characteristic of the specialized and magnet hospital units than of the general medical units. The only indicator that did not discriminate between specialized AIDS units and conventional general medical units was the global clinical environment scale.

Author(s): Baggs, J. G., & Schmitt, M. H.
Article Title: Nurses' and resident physicians' perceptions of the process of collaboration in an MICU
Journal Title: *Research in Nursing & Health*
Volume (Issue): 20(1)   **Year:** 1997 (February)   **Pages:** 71–80

Summary: This qualitative study was designed to investigate care providers' perceptions of the process of nurse–physician collaboration. The sample consisted of 20 participants (10 nurses and 10 residents) from the MICU of an urban university teaching hospital. Two major processes were required to get to the point where the core of the process, working together, could take place: being available and being receptive. Both nurse and resident participants reported only beneficial outcomes from the process of collaboration. Generally the model for working together/collaborating was the same for nurses and residents. The residents focused on strains in the MICU rotation, physical exhaustion, lack of opportunity to be alone, and their multiple patient responsibilities. They wanted nurses to be aware of and sensitive to those concerns. Thus, nurses might believe they were having a collaborative interaction when the resident perceived the same discussion as intrusive or insensitive. The power disparity between the nurses and residents also could have influenced perceptions of collaboration.

Author(s): Clark, L. R., Fraaza, V., Schroeder, S., & Maddens, M. E.
Article Title: Alternative nursing environments: Do they affect hospital outcomes?
Journal Title: *Journal of Gerontological Nursing*
Volume (Issue): 21(11)   **Year:** 1995 (November)   **Pages:** 32–38

Summary: A dayroom program focused intensively on functional needs and was implemented for confused geriatric inpatients who otherwise might have been restrained or required sitters. There were fewer complications from hospitalization documented for dayroom patients. There was an increase in family satisfaction regarding the nursing care provided for patients in the alternative environment.

Author(s): Grindel, C. G., Peterson, K., Kinneman, M., & Turner, T. L.
Article Title: The Practice Environment Project: A process for outcome evaluation
Journal Title: *Journal of Nursing Administration*
Volume (Issue): 26(5)   **Year:** 1996 (May)   **Pages:** 43–51

Summary: The Practice Environment Project (PEP) was created to provide a framework for current and ongoing evaluation of the practice environment. In part 1, quantitative data were collected from nursing staff members (job satisfaction, collaboration with physicians, autonomy), physicians (quality of nursing care, collaboration with nurses), and patients (satisfaction with nursing care). In part 2, focus groups were held with nursing personnel to discuss factors that affected the provision of services. Unit-based action plans were developed to manage barriers to the delivery of services. Patients and physicians reported a high degree of satisfaction with patient care. Physicians reported a higher level of collaboration with nurses than that reported by nurses. Nurses reported a high degree of autonomy in practice; however, in other areas of job satisfaction (development and recognition), they suggested areas for improvement. The PEP created a mechanism to evaluate the current state-of-the-practice environment by identifying core elements for evaluation of work redesign. It also provided a framework for managing barriers that disrupted the delivery of patient care services.

Author(s): Leppa, C. J.
Article Title: Nurse relationships and work group disruption
Journal Title: *Journal of Nursing Administration*
Volume (Issue): 26(10)   **Year:** 1996 (October)   **Pages:** 23–27

Summary: As nursing administrators and managers respond to health care reform pressures with downsizing, rightsizing, and work group reorganization, they need to pay attention to and support the nursing work group relationships. A study of 908 RNs in a variety of nursing work environments in four hospitals indicates that interpersonal relationships are an important part of job satisfaction. There is a relationship between some types of work group disruption and RN satisfaction with interpersonal relationships, and there is a relationship between work group disruption and RN perceptions of patient safety/quality of care.

Author(s): Leveck, M. L., & Jones, C. B.
Article Title: The nursing practice environment, staff retention, and quality of care
Journal Title: *Research in Nursing & Health*
Volume (Issue): 19(4)   **Year:** 1996 (August)   **Pages:** 331–343

Summary: Questionnaire packets were distributed to 670 staff nurses. Nurses were asked to respond based on their perceptions of the work unit. Several instruments were included in the packet to measure the practice environment, including the Group Cohesion Scale, Job Stress Scale, Organizational Work Satisfaction Scale, Nursing Job Satisfaction Scale, and others. The findings point to several important issues related to working conditions and the practice environment, and provide direction for developing strategies to address these concerns. First, units where nurses perceived a participative management style reported higher levels of group cohesion and lower levels of job stress; decreased job stress was found to increase quality of nursing care. Second, participative management also explained nurses' perception of organizational job satisfaction at the unit level. Third, nurses employed on medical-surgical units perceived higher levels of job stress than nurses employed on other types of specialty units. Fourth, the theoretical model helps explain staff nurse retention and quality of care and provides insight into the complex nature of these variables. Staff retention was explained by two factors: experience on the unit and professional job satisfaction.

Author(s): Malloch, K.
Article Title: Healing models for organizations: Description, measurement, and outcomes
Journal Title: *Journal of Healthcare Management*
Volume (Issue): 45(5)   **Year:** 2000 (September–October)   **Pages:** 332–346

Summary: This article describes a study that was developed in response to the increasing work in humanistic or healing environment models and the need for validation of the advantages of such models. A descriptive correlational survey design was used to explore relationships between overall job satisfaction and staff (= 192) perceptions. The authors examined the extent to which the healing model incorporates (1) common understandings of health as a function of body-mind-spirit interrelationships, (2) patient-centered relationships that are caring focused, and (3) a culture supportive of personal growth and mastery. Case study time-series analysis methods were also used to examine trends in organizational performance and comparison of performance to regional norms. The healthy organization model, a framework for health care organizations that incorporates humanistic healing values within the traditional structure, was presented as a result of the study. This model addresses the importance of optimal clinical services, financial performance, and staff satisfaction.

Author(s): Van Ess Coeling, H., & Cukr, P. L.
Article Title: Communication styles that promote perceptions of collaboration, quality, and nurse satisfaction
Journal Title: *Aspens Advisor for Nurse Executives*
Volume (Issue): 15(11)   **Year:** 2000 (August)   **Pages:** 1–12

Summary: The goal of this study was to increase understanding of nurse–physician collaborations. The study used a posttest design with nonequivalent groups to identify whether usage or nonusage of specific communication behaviors were associated with collaboration and its attributed outcomes of improved quality of care and increased nurse satisfaction. A major finding from this study is that usage of an attentive style and avoidance of a contentious or dominant style made a significant difference in the nurses' perceptions of the outcomes.

Perceptions of Quality (N = 20)

Author(s): Bantz, D., Wieseke, A., & Horowitz, J.
Article Title: 2,000 patients relate their hospital experiences
Journal Title: *Nursing Economics*
Volume (Issue): 13(6)   **Year:** 1995   **Pages:** 362–366

Summary: Perspectives of nurses working in seven hospitals across the United States are described. Most nurses believe that all people should have equal access and quality of health care. However, most nurses are unwilling to pay more taxes or donate time to achieve these goals.

Author(s): Harrison, E.
Article Title: Nurse caring and the new health care paradigm
Journal Title: *Journal of Nursing Care Quality*
Volume (Issue): 9(4)   **Year:** 1995 (July)   **Pages:** 14–23

Summary: The current health care environment has ignited a renewed interest in the value of nurse caring and its potential effects on quality of care and patient satisfaction. This study compared perceptions of nurse caring behaviors of inpatient hospice nurses and the families of inpatient hospice clients. The Professional Caring Behaviors Instrument was administered to staff nurses and family representative in the hospice of a Midwestern hospital. Perceptions of nurse caring behaviors were similar for both groups. Only one item, "The caring nurse respects the patient's spiritual beliefs," was significantly more important to the nurses than the family members. Several differences in perceptions were noted in relationship to age.

Author(s): Gray, B. S.
Article Title: Focus group feedback from breast cancer patients
Journal Title: *Journal for Healthcare Quality*
Volume (Issue): 19(5)   **Year:** 1997   **Pages:** 32–36

Summary: A focus group of women with breast cancer was conducted to elicit feedback from clients. Aspects of interest included screening and detection, diagnostic evaluation, treatment, life after cancer, and general perceptions of cancer care. The findings revealed that participants felt the community offered high-quality progressive cancer care. Opportunities for improvement along the continuum were identified, including a need for personalized breast self-exam education, consideration of bed placement in the room following breast surgery, and additional support for breast cancer victims and their husbands. A multidisciplinary plan was developed to address the identified issues.

Author(s): Hostutler, J. J., Taft, S. H., & Snyder, C.
Article Title: Patient needs in the emergency department
Journal Title: *Journal of Nursing Administration*
Volume (Issue): 29(1)   **Year:** 1999 (January)   **Pages:** 43–50

Summary: The purpose of this study was to determine whether ED patients and nurses had similar perceptions of patients' needs, and which needs patients identified as most important. A convenience sample of patients ($n = 126$) and nurses ($n = 49$) in a two-hospital system was used, representing an overall return rate of 31%. *T*-tests and analyses of responses to open-ended questions indicated that nurses may not always perceive accurately patients' needs or the strength of those needs.

Author(s): Hunter, M. A., & Larrabee, J. H.
Article Title: Women's perceptions of quality and benefits of postpartum care
Journal Title: *Journal of Nursing Care Quality*
Volume (Issue): 13(2)   **Year:** 1998 (December)   **Pages:** 21–30

Summary: Increased competition in the United States has led to increased interest in women's perceptions of their obstetric experience. Family-centered postpartum care (FCPPC) was originated to improve women's perceptions of care quality. This study examined differences in and the hypothesized relationship between quality and beneficence in a group receiving traditional postpartum care (TPPC) and a group receiving FCPPC in a safety-net hospital in west Tennessee. Both groups had high mean quality and beneficence scores; however, the FCPPC group's scores were significantly higher than those of the TPPC group. There was a relationship between quality and beneficence for the combined sample. The findings suggest that nurses should incorporate FCPPC approaches as a means of improving perceived quality and benefits.

Author(s): Jones, K. R., Burney, R. E., & Christy, B.
Article Title: Patient expectations for surgery: Are they being met?
Journal Title: *Journal on Quality Improvement*
Volume (Issue): 26(6)   **Year:** 2000   **Pages:** 349–360

Summary: Patients' initial expectations could be categorized as "cure" or "health" outcomes; having less pain, getting better. It was only after surgery that patients identified their undeclared "care" expectations—based on their latent or normative expectations that they would be well cared for, that the system would provide the necessary information, and that the processes of care would meet certain standards.

Author(s): Kangas, S., Kee, C. C., & McKee-Waddle, R.
Article Title: Organizational factors, nurses' job satisfaction, and patient satisfaction with nursing care
Journal Title: *Journal of Nursing Administration*
Volume (Issue): 29(1)   **Year:** 1999 (January)   **Pages:** 32–41

Summary: This study explored differences and relationships among the job satisfaction of RNs, patient satisfaction with nursing care, nursing care delivery models, organizational structure, and organizational culture. As series of instruments were completed by a selected sample of nurses ($n = 92$) and patients ($n = 90$) from three hospitals representing different nursing care models (team nursing, case management, and primary nursing). No differences were found in nurse's job satisfaction or patient satisfaction with nursing care across the three hospitals. A supportive environment was most important to nurses' job satisfaction.

Author(s): Kirchhoff, K. T., & Beckstrand, R. L.
Article Title: Critical care nurses' perceptions of obstacles and helpful behaviors in providing end-of-life care to dying patients
Journal Title: *American Journal of Critical Care*
Volume (Issue): 9(2)   **Year:** 2000 (March)   **Pages:** 96–105

Summary: A questionnaire was mailed to 300 members of the American Association of Critical-Care Nurses to determine the importance of various obstacles and helps in providing end-of-life care as perceived by critical care nurses. Nurses were asked to rate obstacles and helps in giving end-of-life care, provide additional obstacles and/or helps, and answer demographic questions. Six of the top 10 obstacles were related to issues with patients' families that make care at the end of life more difficult. Added obstacles related mostly to problems with physicians' behavior. Most helps were ways to make dying easier for patients and patients' families, such as agreement among physicians about care, dying with dignity, and families' acceptance of the prognosis.

Author(s): Lynn, M. R., & McMillen, B. J.
Article Title: Do nurses know what patients think is important in nursing care?
Journal Title: *Journal of Nursing Care Quality*
Volume (Issue): 13(5)   **Year:** 1999 (June)   **Pages:** 65–74

Summary: For a nurse to provide quality care, she or he must know what patients expect from the nurse. Previous research regarding nurses' insight into patients' expectations of care have been based on idiosyncratic instruments or instruments that measure the perspective of the provider, not the patient. Using the 90 items from the Patient's Perception of Quality Scale—Acute Care Version, an instrument developed from qualitative interviews of patients, 448 patients and 350 nurses from the medical-surgical units in seven hospitals ranked the items, patients from their perspective and nurses as they perceived patients would rank them. Although the rank order of items was similar across patients and nurses, nurses consistently underestimated the extent to which patients valued most aspects of good nursing care.

Author(s): Lynn, M. R., & Moore, K.
Article Title: Relationship between traditional quality indicators and perceptions of care
Journal Title: *Seminars for Nurse Managers*
Volume (Issue): 5(4)   **Year:** 1997 (December)   **Pages:** 187–193

Summary: A study was undertaken to examine the relationships between patients' perceptions of care received, nurses' perceptions of care delivered, and traditional measures of nursing care quality. Findings suggest that traditional quality indicators used in hospitals across the country have little in common with either patients' or nurses' perceptions of quality of care.

Author(s): Niedz, B. A.
Article Title: Correlates of hospitalized patients' perceptions of service quality

Journal Title: *Research in Nursing & Health*
Volume (Issue): 21(4)   **Year:** 1998 (August)   **Pages:** 339–349

Summary: The purpose of this study was to examine patients' perceptions of service quality in relation to four independent variables: (a) nurses' perceptions of human resources practices, (b) nurses' perceptions of autonomy in practice, (c) patient satisfaction with nursing care, and (d) patients' perceptions of organizational climate for service. A sample of 102 nurse–patient dyads was obtained. The first hypothesis predicting a positive relationship between human resource practices as perceived by nurses and service quality as perceived by patients was not supported. The second hypothesis predicting a positive relationship between autonomy in practice as perceived by nurses and service quality as perceived by patients also was not supported. The third hypothesis predicting a positive relationship between patient satisfaction with nursing care and service quality as perceived by patients was supported. The fourth hypothesis predicting a positive relationship between organizational climate for service and service quality as perceived by patients also was supported.

Author(s): O'Connor, S. J., Trinh, H. Q., & Shewchuk, R. M.
Article Title: Perceptual gaps in understanding patient expectations for health care service quality
Journal Title: *Health Care Management Review*
Volume (Issue): 25(2)   **Year:** 2000 (Spring)   **Pages:** 7–23

Summary: This article assesses how well physicians, health administrators, patient-contact employees, and especially medical and nursing students understand patient expectations for service quality as measured by the SERVQUAL scale. Using a cross-sectional research design and discriminant analysis, it was found that health administrators were most likely to accurately estimate the service expectations of patients, and medical and nursing students were most likely to underestimate them.

Author(s): Owens, R., & Cronin, S. N.
Article Title: Nurses' attitudes towards cost-effectiveness and quality of care
Journal Title: *Cost & Quality Quarterly Journal*
Volume (Issue): 4(3)   **Year:** 1998 (October)   **Pages:** 18–22

Summary: A comparative, descriptive design was used to describe nurses' attitudes toward cost effectiveness in nursing practice and its perceived effects on quality of care, and to examine the influence of role, education, and experience on these attitudes. The Blaney Hobson Nursing Attitude Scale was used to measure nurses' attitudes toward cost effectiveness. Scores ranged from 30 to 96, with a mean score of 65.57 (SD = 13.58). Nurses with greater than 10 years of experience had more positive attitudes than nurses with 10 years or less experience. Nurses in administration/management positions had more positive attitudes than did staff nurses. No significant correlation was found between education level and attitudes toward cost effectiveness. The major concern of participants was that quality of care would suffer due to cost containment efforts. The majority of participants agreed that education in cost containment and budgetary issues should begin in basic nursing school and should be included in employer orientation programs.

Author(s): Radwin, L.
Article Title: Oncology patients' perceptions of quality nursing care
Journal Title: *Research in Nursing & Health*
Volume (Issue): 23(3)   Year: 2000 (June)   Pages: 179–190

Summary: The purpose of this grounded theory study was to identify, describe, and analyze theoretically the construct of "quality nursing care" from the patient's perspective. Twenty-two oncology patients composed the purposive sample of informants. Each semistructured interview lasted from 1 to 1.5 hours. The interviews were audiotaped and transcribed. The constant comparative method was used for data analysis. The central construct of the analysis was quality nursing care as seen from the oncology patient's perspective. According to the analysis, two broad outcomes resulted from quality nursing care: a sense of well-being and increased fortitude. According to the analysis, excellent nursing care was characterized by eight attributes: professional knowledge, continuity, attentiveness, coordination, partnership, individualization, rapport, and caring. The eight attributes of quality care detailed in these findings could be considered health care system characteristics actualized by nurses and deemed important by the oncology patients.

Author(s): Radwin, L., & Alster, K.
Article Title: Outcomes of perceived quality nursing care reported by oncology patients
Journal Title: *Scholarly Inquiry for Nursing Practice*
Volume (Issue): 13(4)   Year: 1999 (Winter)   Pages: 327–343, 345–347

Summary: At a time when health care quality is being defined by providers, administrators, and third-party payers, it is more important than ever to ensure that patients' voices are heard. Patients can tell us not only what makes nursing care excellent; they can tell us how this care makes a difference. This article reports on the outcomes ascribed to quality nursing care by a group of purposively selected oncology patients who participated in a grounded theory study. One outcome was a sense of well-being comprising trust, optimism, and authenticity. A second outcome, increased fortitude, occurred when the patients felt that they had the readiness, strength, and stamina to undergo cancer treatment and bear its effects. The outcomes are described and discussed in relation to existing scholarly work.

Author(s): Richmond, I., & Roberson, E.
Article Title: The customer is always right: Patients' perceptions of psychiatric nursing actions
Journal Title: *Journal of Nursing Care Quality*
Volume (Issue): 9(2)   Year: 1995   Pages: 36–43

Summary: This study examined psychiatric inpatients' ($N = 100$) perceptions of interactions with health care providers as a factor in assessing the quality of care provided in the setting of a large urban medical center. Fifty commonly used psychiatric nursing actions were evaluated by patients. Significant differences were found between the general psychiatric patient population and the substance abuse population in perception of helpfulness and frequency of performance with 7 of 50 nursing actions.

Author(s): Rosenfeld, P., Duthie, E., Bier, J., Bowar-Ferres, S., Fulmer, T., Iervolino, L., McClure, M. L., McGivern, D. O., & Roncoli, M.
Article Title: Engaging staff nurses in evidence-based research to identify nursing practice problems and solutions
Journal Title: *Applied Nursing Research*
Volume (Issue): 13(4)   **Year:** 2000 (November)   **Pages:** 197–203

Summary: The research model incorporated both survey and focus group methods used by nursing leaders in administration and practice to identify and prioritize nursing research and clinical needs in their organizations. The goal was to establish consensus among clinicians and researchers about significant issues in the institution requiring in-depth attention. A second objective was to design a survey instrument that is easy to complete and could be distributed, collected, and analyzed easily, thereby providing empirical data to the clinicians in a timely manner and in a simple format. This expedited process enabled specific action plans to be developed around the identified problems. Moreover, the process promoted interest in advancing nursing research and evidence-based practice among the clinicians and administrators.

Author(s): Sales, A., Lurie, N., Moscovice, I., & Goes, J.
Article Title: Is quality in the eye of the beholder?
Journal Title: *The Joint Commission Journal on Quality Improvement*
Volume (Issue): 21(5)   **Year:** 1995   **Pages:** 219–225

Summary: In late 1992, 669 hospital administrators, QA coordinators, physicians, and nurses from 72 hospitals in six states were surveyed by telephone. Respondents were asked to identify the most serious issue related to quality of care in their hospital. Of all the respondents, hospital administrators were most likely to identify quality issues related to organizational/institutional issues. QA coordinators, most of whom had nursing backgrounds, were most likely to identify organizational and patient care issues. Physician responses were distributed approximately evenly across issues related to physicians, the organization, and patient care. Nurses were most likely to identify issues related to patient care and patient satisfaction. The findings validate the viewpoint that quality is in the eye of the beholder and that surveys that specifically target certain disciplinary groups may yield important information about issues related to quality care.

Author(s): Williams, S. A.
Article Title: Quality and care: Patients' perceptions
Journal Title: *Journal of Nursing Care Quality*
Volume (Issue): 12(6)   **Year:** 1998 (August)   **Pages:** 18–25, 70–72

Summary: Patients and health care professionals view quality nursing care from different perspectives. Health care professionals view competent nursing care as quality nursing care. Patients perceive quality nursing care as caring, inter-personal interactions. Institutions measure quality care through satisfaction surveys that exclude components of nurse caring behaviors. In three studies utilizing the Holistic Caring Inventory (HCI), patients perceived nurse caring behaviors and attitudes that indicated quality nursing care. The way to bridge the gap between institutions' and patients' perceptions of quality care lies in valuing the interactions that patients consider quality care and including these interactions in measures of quality care.

Author(s): Young, W. B., Minnick, A. F., & Marcantonio, R.
Article Title: How wide is the gap in defining quality care? Comparison of patient and nurse perceptions of important aspects of patient care
Journal Title: *Journal of Nursing Administration*
Volume (Issue): 26(5)   **Year:** 1996 (May)   **Pages:** 15–20

Summary: Two thousand fifty-one medical-surgical patients, 1264 staff members, and 97 nurse-managers from 17 randomly selected hospitals participated in study activities related to selected aspects of patient care. Trained interviewers surveyed patients by telephone within 26 days of discharge using a pretested instrument. Staff members and managers completed a coordinated written tool. Staff members perceive correctly that patients value differently various aspects of care but do not agree with their managers on patients' values of aspects of care. Unit staff members' and managers' beliefs regarding patients' care values did not match those of their patients. A unit's errors in defining patients' values may be self-reinforcing. Strategies to reorient personnel may help to bridge the gap and change practice.

Patient/Caregiver Satisfaction (N = 15)

Author(s): Bailey, D. A., & Mion, L. C.
Article Title: Improving care givers' satisfaction with information received during hospitalization
Journal Title: *Journal of Nursing Administration*
Volume (Issue): 27(1)   **Year:** 1997   **Pages:** 21–27

Summary: As competition for patient volume escalates among hospital providers, administrators must identify ways to attract new patients and maintain or increase patient volume. Family caregivers are known to greatly influence individuals' choices in these maters of selection of health care services and providers. The results of a successful nurse-initiated daily phone call program, designed to improve family caregiver satisfaction by enhancing the provision of patient-specific information, are presented. The components of the program, associated costs, and implications on delivery of care are discussed.

Author(s): Bruce, T. A., Bowman, J. M., & Brown, S. T.
Article Title: Factors that influence patient satisfaction in the emergency department
Journal Title: *Journal of Nursing Care Quality*
Volume (Issue): 13(2)   **Year:** 1998 (December)   **Pages:** 31–37

Summary: This descriptive correlation study examined the satisfaction levels of urgent and nonurgent patients in relation to nursing care, the EDenvironment, ancillary services, and information received. The sample consisted of 28 subjects, with the majority of patients being very satisfied with nursing care. The primary area of concern was information about the length of waiting time. The satisfaction levels of ED patients with the care they receive has become increasingly important in today's health care environment. ED nurses play an important role in ensuring that patients are satisfied and receive quality care.

Author(s): Blackington, S. M., & McLauchlan, T.
Article Title: Continuous quality improvement in the neonatal intensive care unit: Evaluating parent satisfaction.
Journal Title: *Journal of Nursing Care Quality*
Volume (Issue): 9(4)   **Year:** 1995   **Pages:** 78–85

Summary: A comprehensive approach to the delivery of family-centered care in the NICU requires that parental perceptions of care giving be addressed. The Parent Feedback Questionnaire is based on researched needs of NICU parents. Specific dimensions of needs (informational, emotional, parenting, and environmental) and overall satisfaction are identified and included in survey items. Ongoing feedback from parents is obtained and incorporated into a planned multidisciplinary CQI program. Evaluation of data has resulted in planned interventions to reduce sources of stress and dissatisfaction for parents.

Author(s): Clark, C. A., Pokorny, M. E., & Brown, S. T.
Article Title: Consumer satisfaction with nursing care in a rural community hospital emergency department
Journal Title: *Journal of Nursing Care Quality*
Volume (Issue): 10(2)   **Year:** 1996   **Pages:** 49–57

Summary: The article describes a study undertaken to assess patient satisfaction with nursing care in a rural hospital ED with respect to psychological safety, discharge teaching, information giving, and technical competence. This descriptive research utilized Davis' Consumer Emergency Care Satisfaction Scale to determine the degree to which 52 patients perceived overall satisfaction with nursing care. Findings indicated that patients were satisfied with nursing care. No statistically significant effect of gender or education level on consumer satisfaction or on any subscale was detected, but African-American consumers were less satisfied with discharge teaching, which may suggest that discharge teaching should reflect the cultural diversity of consumers presenting to the ED. Nursing staff may need to spend more time with rural African-American consumers. Staff may need to be inserviced to meet the cultural and educational needs of African-Americans.

Author(s): Haynie, L., & Garrett, B.
Article Title: Developing a customer-service and cost-effectiveness team
Journal Title: *Journal for Healthcare Quality*
Volume (Issue): 21(6)   **Year:** 1999   **Pages:** 28–34

Summary: This article describes the development of a "resource team " to improve customer service scores, system efficiency, and staff accountability in a health care organization in northeast Georgia. Another goal of the team was to maintain an emphasis on cost-effective and efficient utilization of resources. One-year following implementation customer satisfaction scores were reported to be in the top third for inpatient services in a database of 19 other hospitals, a rating of third-highest for emergency services in a database of 28 other hospitals, and a benchmark rating for outpatient services in the fourth quarter of 1998. The authors conclude that, although customer satisfaction scores were not as high as the organization wanted, the improvements are indicators of a positive culture change.

Author(s): Jacox, A. K., Bausell, B. R., & Mahrenholz, D. M.
Article Title: Patient satisfaction with nursing care in hospitals
Journal Title: *Outcomes Management for Nursing Practice*
Volume (Issue): 1(1)   **Year:** 1997 (October–December)   **Pages:** 20–28

Summary: This article reports on two preliminary studies and one major study of the Patient Satisfaction with Nursing Care Questionnaire. This questionnaire includes four general questions related to the patient's satisfaction with the overall stay in the hospital, food provided, and medical and nursing care received and 15 items that measure satisfaction with three dimensions of nursing care: caring about patients (interpersonal), technical skills, and patient education.

Author(s): Kellar, N., Martinez, J., Finnis, N., Bolger, A. & von Gunten, C. F.
Article Title: Characterization of an acute impatient hospice palliative care unit in a U.S. teaching hospital
Journal Title: *Journal of Nursing Administration*
Volume (Issue): 26(3) **Year:** 1996 (March) **Pages:** 16–20

Summary: The purpose of this study was to identify current uses of an existing hospice palliative care inpatient care unit in an academic medical center setting and to determine whether the high level of satisfaction among family members, as perceived by the staff, was accurate. Prospective assessment of 100 consecutive unit admissions in 1993 revealed a patient population with more diversity than originally planned for this unit. Results of family and patient satisfaction surveys ($n = 92$) indicated that the "vast majority" of respondents believed that the move to the palliative care unit was important, and that the care received was important and different from that in other settings. Superior, professional nursing care; security for family when they could not be at the bedside; a warm, home-like environment; large rooms; relaxed visiting hours; and the attention given to families were cited as "advantages of the unit." Added helps included allowing music, pets, and so forth into the patient's room. Nurses do not acknowledge having difficulty providing care to dying patients aside from conflicts that arise because of patients' families and physicians.

Author(s): Koman, A. R., Kunik, M. E., Molinari, V., Ponce, H., Rezabek, P., & Orengo, C. A.
Article Title: Discharge plans from a geropsychiatric unit: Patient and family satisfaction
Journal Title: *Clinical Gerontologist*
Volume (Issue): 20(4) **Year:** 1999 **Pages:** 29–38

Summary: Satisfaction with discharge placement and factors contributing to that satisfaction were rated by 80 patients and/or their primary caregiver within 1 month of discharge. Participants were generally highly satisfied with the time and effort spent by the treatment team (83%) and about half considered themselves very involved in discharge planning. Among those discharged to home ($n = 44$), the factors most commonly associated with satisfaction were the availability of familiar caregivers (73%) and familiar environment (68%). The most common factors associated with satisfaction with discharge to a nursing home ($n = 33$) were more care provided (75.8%) and more caregivers available (81.8%). Among the participants discharged to home, the factor most commonly associated with dissatisfaction was high cost (7%). Factors associated with dissatisfaction with discharge to a nursing home included unfamiliar environment (24%) and high cost (21%).

Author(s): Raper, J. L.
Article Title: A cognitive approach to patient satisfaction with emergency department nursing care
Journal Title: *Journal of Nursing Care Quality*
Volume (Issue): 10(4) **Year:** 1996 (July) **Pages:** 48–58

Summary: The assessment of patient satisfaction is an integral part of any quality improvement activity. In this study, patient satisfaction with ED nursing care was significantly positively related to the patient's self-perceived improvement and to the patient's admission to the hospital. Patient satisfaction with ED nursing care was not significantly related to patient acuity or other individual patient differences (age, gender, marital status, length of stay, type of treatment, number of previous ED visits, race, payer source, pain, or presence of chronic health problems). Psychological safety and information giving were found to contribute significantly to patient satisfaction with the ED nurse. Patient satisfaction with ED nursing care contributed significantly to the patients' intention to return to the ED.

Author(s): Raper, J., Davis, B. A., & Scott, L.
Article Title: Patient satisfaction with emergency department triage nursing care: A multicenter study
Journal Title: *Journal of Nursing Care Quality*
Volume (Issue): 13(6)   **Year:** 1999 (August)   **Pages:** 11–24

Summary: This descriptive, correlational study examines relationships between individual patient and nurse characteristics, and patient satisfaction with triage and ED nursing care. The convenience sample consisted of Urgent/Delayed patients ($N = 378$) triaged in an urban academic medical center. Analysis of variance revealed significantly higher levels of patient satisfaction at the academic medical center, whereas higher levels of intent to return were reported by subjects from the Catholic-affiliated hospital. Educational preparation of the triage nurse was identified as a significant predictor of both patient satisfaction with triage nursing care and loyalty to a specific hospital.

Author(s): Schaffer, P., Vaughn, G., Kenner, C., Donohue, F., & Longo, A.
Article Title: Revision of a parent satisfaction survey based on the parent perspective
Journal Title: *Journal of Pediatric Nursing: Nursing Care of Children & Families*
Volume (Issue): 15(6)   **Year:** 2000 (December)   **Pages:** 373–377

Summary: The Parent Satisfaction Survey at a 250-bed children's hospital was revised based on what parents thought was most important for a nurse to do for themselves and their children. This report is based on a retrospective review of 1405 self-reported parent surveys collected as a performance improvement activity over 12 months. Surveys were distributed to parents of hospitalized children and were returned anonymously to mailboxes on the units. Using content analysis, a group of pediatric nurses reviewed the parents' comments to determine major themes. The themes were caring, communication, safety, environment, and appreciation. The parent survey was revised to include the themes parents identified as important.

Author(s): Silberzweig, J., & Giguere, B.
Article Title: Redesign for patient satisfaction
Journal Title: *Journal of Nursing Care Quality*
Volume (Issue): 11(2)   **Year:** 1996 (December)   **Pages:** 25–33

Summary: In this era of changing health care systems, the word redesign is often linked with mergers, layoffs, or an economic move to balance the bottom line. Redesign is often perceived as a way to reduce the need for professional nurses by eliminating job functions. In this cost-cutting milieu, however, the most important factor—the patient—has been put aside. The article explores what factors contribute to patient satisfaction and describes the redesign process that was implemented at one institution to increase patients' satisfaction during hospitalization.

Author(s): VanderVeen, L., & Ritz, M.
Article Title: Customer satisfaction: A practical approach for hospitals
Journal Title: *Journal for Healthcare Quality*
Volume (Issue): 18(2)   **Year:** 1996 (March/April)   **Pages:** 10–15

Summary: A California hospital developed a program to better serve and satisfy its customers. This article details the hospital's plan to implement the program with the collection and use of data to measure success, promote staff accountability, and, ultimately, demonstrate improved customer satisfaction as measured by fewer complaints. The various activities initiated to promote staff education and recognize employees also are briefly addressed.

Author(s): Williams, S. A.
Article Title: The relationship of patients' perceptions of holistic nurse caring to satisfaction with nursing care
Journal Title: *Journal of Nursing Care Quality*
Volume (Issue): 11(5)   **Year:** 1997 (June)   **Pages:** 15–29

Summary: Hospitalized patients interact with nurses more often than with other health care providers. Qualitative studies have identified patients' and nurses' perceptions of nursing care behaviors. Few studies have explored nurse caring behavior in relation to patient satisfaction. The article describes a study designed to determine whether there is a relationship between patients' perceptions of nurse caring and satisfaction with nursing care and whether selected patient variables significantly affect that relationship. In the patient population studied, after controlling for patient variables of age, gender, and level of pain, a significant positive relationship was found between patients' perceptions of nurse caring and their satisfaction with nursing care.

Author(s): Wolf, Z. R., Colahan M., Costello, A., Warwick, F., Ambrose, M. S., & Giardino, E. R.
Article Title: Research utilization. Relationship between nurse caring and patient satisfaction
Journal Title: *MEDSURG Nursing*
Volume (Issue): 7(2)   **Year:** 1998 (April)   **Pages:** 99–105

Summary: A correlational study examined patients' ($n = 335$) reports of nurse caring and satisfaction with nursing care, using the Caring Behaviors Inventory and Patient Satisfaction Instrument. A strong, positive correlation ($r = .78$, $p < .001$, $r^2 = 61.46\%$) was found. The outcomes of this study have important implications for adult health nurses.

Technology Use (N = 3)

Author(s): Chewitt, M. D., Fallis, W. M., & Suski, M. C.
Article Title: The surgical hotline: Bridging the gap between hospital and home
Journal Title: *Journal of Nursing Administration*
Volume (Issue): 27(12)   **Year:** 1997 (December)   **Pages:** 42–49

Summary: This article describes the development, implementation, and evaluation of a surgical hotline designed to provide a continuum of care to postsurgical patients. Data for the 4-month evaluation period were collected through analysis of data collections sheet and through patient (n = 100) and staff (n = 17) satisfaction surveys. Patient perceptions of the surgical hotline were positive (85%), and staff perceptions were generally positive. Eleven of the nurses felt that the hotline was overly time consuming, but the same number felt it was a service important enough to continue.

Author(s): Henzler, C., & Harper, J.
Article Title: Implementing a computer-assisted appropriateness review using DRG 182/183
Journal Title: *The Joint Commission Journal on Quality Improvement*
Volume (Issue): 21(5)   **Year:** 1995   **Pages:** 239–247

Summary: One hospital undertook to redesign the process of appropriateness reviews using a computer-assisted methodology. The change was predicated on accessing electronically recorded clinical data collected as part of a state-mandated discharge reporting requirement. More than 90% of DRG 182/183 (gastrointestinal/esophagitis) admissions were deemed appropriate on the basis of later manual reviews. This redesign was accomplished at no added expense, and the amount of time required to complete the study was decreased. The ability to easily examine relationships identified during the evaluation was also expanded. The experience led to greater enthusiasm on the part of the medical staff to pursue more quality improvement projects.

Author(s): Nahm, R., & Poston, I.
Article Title: Measurement of the effects of an integrated, point-of-care computer system on quality of nursing documentation and patient satisfaction
Journal Title: *Computers in Nursing*
Volume (Issue): 18(5)   **Year:** 2000 (September–October)   **Pages:** 220–229

Summary: This quasi-experimental, modified time series study measured the effects of the nursing module of a point-of-care clinical information system on nursing documentation and patient satisfaction. Measurements were taken before implementation of the module and at 6-, 12-, and 18-month intervals postimplementation. Quality of nursing documentation was measured by compliance to items applicable to nursing documentation selected from the JCAHO Closed Medical Review Tool. Patient satisfaction was measured by using the Risser Patient Satisfaction Scale. The study data showed a statistically significant increase in the quality of nursing documentation after implementation of the computerized nursing documentation system, as well as a decrease in variability in charting, as evidenced by a decrease in standard deviations. A significant increase in charting compliance was still occurring between the 12- and the 18-month time points after initiation of automated documentation. The point-of-care computer system did not seem to affect patient satisfaction with the nurse–patient relationship.

Patient Education (N = 1)

Author(s): Patyk, M., Gaynor, S., & Verdin, J.
Article Title: Patient education resource assessment: Project management
Journal Title: *Journal of Nursing Care Quality*
Volume (Issue): 14(2)   **Year:** 2000 (January)   **Pages:** 14–20

Summary: To thrive in today's health care environment, hospitals are constantly striving to exceed their customers' expectations in delivering quality care in a cost-effective manner. Meeting the patient educational needs of the consumer is one well-recognized aspect of quality care. Delivering quality care does not happen by chance; rather, it requires intense planning. Our academic medical center formalized this process by empowering professional staff from Nursing Development to develop and implement a patient education strategic plan. This article outlines the project management for the assessment phase of this strategic planning process. The findings were instrumental in outlining the future direction for patient education initiatives that will benefit both the patient and the organization.

Veterans Affairs Medical Centers Nursing Quality Measurement Studies

6

Overview

Nursing quality measurement studies conducted within Veterans Affairs Medical Centers (VAMC) during this period were focused on specific clinical issues and quality improvement efforts. One identifiable trend in this setting is that clients entering the VAMC reflect an increasingly older population. The studies included in this review dealt with fall prevention programs, alcohol withdrawal, and case management issues for older adults. In the future, like many long-term care facilities, VAMCs will need to focus on quality of care issues for the older adult. The potential for using the MDS and quality indicators in VAMCs has yet to be realized.

The five Veterans Affairs Medical Centers nursing quality measurement studies in this chapter are organized as follows:

▌ Clinical issues
▌ Quality improvement

Clinical Issues (N = 3)

Author(s): Galindo-Ciocon, D. J., Ciocon, J. O., & Galindo, D. J.
Article Title: Gait training and falls in the elderly
Journal Title: Journal of Gerontological Nursing
Volume (Issue): 21(6)   **Year:** 1995 (June)   **Pages:** 11–17

Summary: Patients with gait and balance disorder, as measured by the Tinetti Mobility Scale, can benefit from physical therapist-assisted gait training. Score in the Tinetti Mobility Scale negatively correlates with the number of recurrence of falls. The nurse's role includes identification of those who are at risk for falls, assessment of their response to training in the prevention of recurrence of falls, and the effect of training on their mobility and independence.

Author(s): Gunn, S., Hanisch, P., & Wood, D.
Article Title: CQI action team: Responding to the detoxification patient
Journal Title: The Joint Commission Journal on Quality Improvement
Volume (Issue): 21(10)   **Year:** 1995   **Pages:** 531–540

Summary: The management of detoxification patients is a complex inter-disciplinary effort requiring involvement, cooperation, and understanding from staff at all levels of the facility. Alcohol-related diagnoses were the highest admission diagnosis at the Veterans Affairs Medical Center (VAMC), yet only 44% of the detoxification patients admitted to the VAMC were placed in beds specifically designed for detoxification. Data analysis of admission and discharge trends, laboratory results, and bed census revealed discrepancies with several widespread myths held by local health care workers. These misperceptions and attitudes often interfered with treatment. Recommended changes included the development of a clinical pathway for the detoxification patient, implementation of an alcohol withdrawal assessment tool to manage and treat the patient at risk for experiencing alcohol withdrawal, and hospital-wide education on management of the detoxification patient.

Author(s): Mosley, A., Galindo-Ciocon, D., Peak, N., & West, M. J.
Article Title: Initiation and evaluation of a research-based fall prevention program
Journal Title: Journal of Nursing Care Quality
Volume (Issue): 13(2)   **Year:** 1998 (December)   **Pages:** 38–44

Summary: This study evaluated the effectiveness of research-based interventions in preventing falls. The interventions were based on research studies, experts' opinions, and a pilot study. Thirteen units (72%) had reduced fall rates. The fall rate 2 years before ($0 = 7.07$; SD = 1.7) and 2 years after ($0 = 6.33$; SD = 1.731) the intervention was significantly different ($p < .003$). Sixteen patients who fell were at risk (fall assessment score = 17.4 ± 5.3) and had a history of falls. The most common site for falls was at the bedside. Most falls occurred during walking, climbing over the siderails, and accidentally rolling out of bed. Thus, a research-based fall prevention is effective in reducing falls.

Quality Improvement (N = 2)

Author(s): Holle, M. L., Rick, C., Sliefert, M. K., & Stephens, K.
Article Title: Integrating patient care delivery
Journal Title: Journal of Nursing Administration
Volume (Issue): 25(7/8)   **Year:** 1995 (July/August)   **Pages:** 32–37

Summary: Concepts of coordinated care, case management, and continuous quality improvement were applied by a medical center nursing service to improve continuity and coordination of patient care between inpatient and outpatient programs. Quality and cost outcomes are presented for a pilot project with a total hip replacement population.

Author(s): Weaver, F. M., Conrad, K. J., Guihan, M., Byck, G. R., Manheim, L. M., & Hughes, S. L.
Article Title: Evaluation of a prospective payment system for VA contract nursing homes
Journal Title: Evaluation & The Health Professions
Volume (Issue): 19(4)   **Year:** 1996 (December)   **Pages:** 423–442

Summary: An evaluation of a pilot program for community nursing home care reimbursement by VAMC was undertaken. Eight VAMCs began using the Enhanced Prospective Payment System (EPPS) in 1992. These sites were compared to eight customary payment sites in a pre-/posttest quasi-experimental design. Outcomes included access to care, administrative workload, quality of care, and cost. As expected, per diem costs were significantly higher for EPPS than customary reimbursement patients. However, EPPS sites placed veterans more quickly than comparison sites and reduced administrative workload associated with placement. EPPS sites also increased the number of Medicare-certified homes under contract and placed significantly more veterans who received therapy. Savings in hospital days more than offset the increased cost of nursing home placement.

Long-Term Care Nursing Quality Measurement Studies

7

Overview

Since 1995, long-term care studies examining quality of care have increased remarkably. In the 1995 review, only nine studies were identified: three focused on quality indicators, four about specific clinical issues, one in organizational factors, and one regarding patient satisfaction. In our review from 1995–2000, a total of 56 studies were identified that examined quality in long-term care. Nine focused on quality measurement specifically, 8 about the nursing home MDS and quality indicators derived from those data, 21 about specific clinical issues, 5 about satisfaction with care, 2 with end-of-life issues, 2 with family involvement in care, and 8 about staffing and quality.

Nurse researchers are directing their efforts on resident outcomes and case-mix adjustment (Anderson, et al., 1999) as well as examining QIs as useful for improving quality of care (Rantz et al., 1996, 1997, 2000a). Clinical issues are increasingly the focus of research, for example, disruptive behaviors (Hoeffer et al., 1997), incontinence (Simmons & Schnelle, 1999), weight loss (Gants, 1997), mealtime experience (Kayser-Jones & Schell, 1997), walking program (Koroknay et al., 1995), and care planning (Cox, 1998). From a broad perspective of quality, nurse-researchers have developed a new instrument to measure care quality in nursing facilities by quickly walking through a facility and observing key sensory indicators (Rantz et al, 2000b).

Important organizational issues of staffing are of concern, are the focus of researcher interest, and are critical to quality in long-term care. The views of nursing assistants are extremely relevant to quality of care (Bowers, Esmond, & Jacobson, 2000). Increasing involvement of registered nurses in participation in decision making improves resident outcomes (Anderson & McDaniel, 1999). Having administrators with nursing backgrounds who spend time involved in patient care positively influences quality of care (Singh et al., 1996). There is a relationship between the ratio of total nursing staff and quality of care as measured by nursing-related deficiencies (Johnson-Pawlson & Infeld, 1996) and fewer registered nurse and nursing assistant hours are associated with total deficiencies and quality of care deficiencies (Harrington et al., 2000).

Consumer (resident) satisfaction has emerged in the last 5 years with five studies identified, four more than the single study identified in the 1995 review. Satisfaction with care is measured from the perspective of the resident (Watson, Mobarack, & Stimson, 1999), the perspectives of the family (Steffen & Nystrom, 1997; Wakefield, Buckwalter & Collins, 1997), and the points of views of both families and residents (Meister & Boyle, 1996; Rantz et al, 1999).

In summary, quality measurement in long-term care is receiving more attention. Perhaps with the aging of our population becoming apparent to the general population and to researchers, the imperative to examine quality of care provided in long-term care is finally coming to the forefront. If this is the case, it is likely that research in this area will continue to grow.

The 55 long-term care nursing quality measurement studies in this chapter are organized as follows:

- Clinical issues
- Quality measurement
- Staffing
- NMDS/quality indicators
- Satisfaction with care
- Family involvement
- End of life

Clinical Issues (N = 21)

Author(s): Berlowitz, D. R., Ash, A. S., Brandeis, G. H., Brand, H. K., Halpern, J. L., & Moskowitz, M. A.
Article Title: Rating long-term care facilities on pressure ulcer development: Importance of case-mix adjustment.
Journal Title: *Annals of Internal Medicine*
Volume (Issue): 124(6)   **Year:** 1996 (March 15)   **Pages:** 557–563

Summary: The purpose of this study was to determine the importance of case-mix adjustment in interpreting differences in rates of pressure ulcer development in long-term care facilities. A sample of 31,150 intermediate medicine and nursing home residents who were initially free of pressure ulcers and were institutionalized between October 1991 and April 1993 was used to derive predictors of pressure ulcer development. The resulting model was validated in a separate sample of 17,946 residents institutionalized from April 1993 to October 1993. Facility-level rates of pressure ulcer development, both unadjusted and adjusted for case mix using the predictive model, were compared. Eleven factors predicted pressure ulcer development.

Author(s): Berlowitz, D. R., Bezerra, H. Q., Brandeis, G. H., Kader, B., & Anderson, J. J.
Article Title: Are we improving the quality of nursing home care: The case of pressure ulcers

Journal Title: *Journal of the American Geriatrics Society*
Volume (Issue): 48(1)   **Year:** 2000 (January)   **Pages:** 59–62

Summary: This study evaluated a large provider of nursing home care to determine whether risk-adjusted rates of pressure ulcer development have changed. The Nursing Minimum Data Set (NMDS) was used to study National Health-Care Corporation nursing homes from 1991 through 1995. Rates of pressure ulcer development were calculated for successive 6-month periods by determining the proportion of residents initially ulcer-free having a stage 2 or larger pressure ulcer on subsequent assessments. Rates were risk adjusted for patient characteristics. The proportion of new ulcers that were deep (stages 3 or 4) were also calculated. Risk-adjusted rates of pressure ulcer development were examined based on 144,379 observations of 30,510 residents at 107 nursing homes. The number of observations per 6-month period ranged from 11,041 to 15,805. Between 1991 and 1995, there was a significant rate decline of more than 25%. Additionally, the proportion of new ulcers that were stages 3 or 4 declined from 30 to 22%. Nursing homes showed significant improvement in the quality of pressure ulcer preventive care from 1991 to 1995.

Author(s): Carrol-Solomon, P. A., Christian, V., Denny, D. S., Nordan, V. N., Therriault, M. F., & Van Wisklen, R.
Article Title: Preserving residents' rights in long-term care settings: A values-based approach to restraint reduction
Journal Title: *Journal for Healthcare Quality*
Volume (Issue): 22(4)   **Year:** 2000 (July/August)   **Pages:** 10–19

Summary: This article describes a knowledge transfer process developed by Catholic Health Ease (CHE), headquartered in Newtown Square, Pennsylvania, and that focuses on one indicator of care, physical restraint use, in the skilled nursing/long-term care setting. The values-based process focuses on preserving residents' rights and using comparative data sharing as the basis for identifying opportunities for improvement. Further, it builds on a collaborative cyclical model employed by all the CHE System's freestanding and hospital-based long-term care facilities. The experiences of four of the system's facilities are described; each demonstrates different aspects of implementing mission-oriented strategies to target restraint reduction.

Author(s): Castle, N. G.
Article Title: Deficiency citations for physical restraint use in nursing homes
Journal Title: *Journals of Gerontology Series B—Psychological Sciences & Social Sciences*
Volume (Issue): 55B(1)   **Year:** 2000 (January)   **Pages:** S33–S40

Summary: This article investigates which structure and process factors of nursing homes are associated with a deficiency citation for restraint use. Nationally representative data from the 1997 On-line Survey Certification of Automated Records are used, first, to provide descriptive analyses, and second, for logistic regression analyses of structure and process factors associated with a deficiency citation for restraint use. A total of 2321 facilities were found to have at least one restraint deficiency citation, and 14,703 had none. After controlling for seven other key variables, five structural factors and six process factors are significant. The structural factors—larger bed size, for-profit ownership, and hospital based—were significantly associated with a higher likelihood of a deficiency citation for restraint use; higher numbers of full-time equivalent specialists per resident and nurse aide training were significantly associated with a lower likelihood. The process factors—suctioning therapy, pain management, and bladder training—were significantly associated with a lower likelihood of a deficiency citation for restraint use; intravenous therapy, higher use of catheters and physical restraints were significantly associated with a higher likelihood of a deficiency citation. This analysis establishes links between structures and processes and the outcome of a deficiency citation for restraint use.

Author(s): Castle, N. G., & Fogel, B.
Article Title: Organizational structure and outcomes for nursing home residents with mental disorders
Journal Title: *Journal of Mental Health & Aging*
Volume (Issue): 4(1)   **Year:** 1998 (Spring)   **Pages:** 105–124

Summary: Persons with mental disorders in nursing homes total almost 1 million. However, there is great variation in the quality of care these residents receive. Using Donabedian's structure, process, and outcome model of quality, this study examines the degree to which organizational structures affect quality outcomes experienced by nursing home residents with mental disorders. Several structural factors are found to be significantly associated with each of the quality outcomes (mood, social engagement, behavioral problems, cognitive performance scale [CPS] scores, activities of daily living [ADL] scores, and mortality) indicating that these mental health outcomes are not solely dependent on resident characteristics.

Author(s): Cox, R. A.
Article Title: Implementing nurse sensitive outcomes into care planning at a long-term care facility
Journal Title: *Journal of Nursing Care Quality*
Volume (Issue): 12(5)   **Year:** 1998 (June)   **Pages:** 41–51

Summary: This article describes one long-term care facility's efforts to implement standardized language in the care planning process. Federal regulations for long-term care mandate the use of a uniform comprehensive assessment tool. Eighteen Resident Assessment Protocols (RAPs) were identified for data collection. Computer databases were revised for care planning. Appropriate North American Nursing Diagnosis Association (NANDA) diagnoses were linked to each RAP. Nursing-Sensitive Outcomes were linked to each NANDA as goals. Nursing Interventions Classifications (NICs) were linked to NANDA diagnosis and nursing-sensitive outcomes as approaches. The databases were illustrated, and frequently used NANDAs and nursing-sensitive outcomes are identified.

Author(s): Gants, R.

Article Title: Detection and correction of underweight problems in nursing home residents

Journal Title: *Journal of Gerontological Nursing*

Volume (Issue): 23(12)   **Year:** 1997 (December)   **Pages:** 26–31

Summary: Excessive weight loss in the elderly is a well-known phenomenon with ramifications that may result in illness and death. In this study, the underweight residents of a long-term care facility were treated with individual nursing care plans based on calorie-rich, low-volume diets and were successful in increasing, or at least stabilizing, their weight and general health level. Nurses can take action in preventing physical deterioration and weight problems by preserving and correcting weight in the elderly.

Author(s): Gibson, C. J., Opalka, P. C., Moore, C. A., Brady, R. S., & Mion, L. C.

Article Title: Effectiveness of bran supplement on the bowel management of elderly rehabilitation patients

Journal Title: *Journal of Gerontological Nursing*

Volume (Issue): 21(10)   **Year:** 1995 (October)   **Pages:** 21–30

Summary: Constipation is a common problem in the elderly that affects up to 20% of those 65 years and older. Patients receiving the fiber supplement had a significantly lower number of bowel agents per day as compared to the control patients. Side effects from the additional fiber occurred in a subgroup of patients; thus, institution of additional fiber to the diets of ill, physically dependent patients is best done gradually and with close monitoring.

Author(s): Hasel, K. L., & Erickson, R. S.

Article Title: Effect of cerumen on infrared ear temperature measurement

Journal Title: *Journal of Gerontological Nursing*

Volume (Issue): 21(12)   **Year:** 1995 (December)   **Pages:** 6–14

Summary: One-third or more of elderly individuals may have occlusive amounts of cerumen in one or both ear canals. In this study, occlusion of the ear canal with cerumen tended to lower ear-based temperature measurements with an infrared thermometer by an average of about 0.2 °F (0.1 °C). Removing cerumen from the ear canal is likely to result in improved hearing as well as more accurate ear-based temperature measurements. Accuracy of ear-based temperature measurements is enhanced by properly positioning the thermometer in the ear canal, taking two readings each time and recording the higher value, using the same ear for repeated measurements, and keeping the probe window clean.

Author(s): Holtzman, J., Degelau, J., Meyers, R., Christianson, C., & Lurie, N.

Article Title: Development and testing of a process measure of nursing home quality of care

Journal Title: *Journal of the American Geriatrics Society*

Volume (Issue): 45(10)   **Year:** 1997 (October)   **Pages:** 1203–1207

Summary: Flowsheets designed to capture the critical elements of care were developed by an expert panel then used to develop and test quality of care process measures for three medical conditions of nursing home patients: fever, shortness of breath, and chest pain. Nursing home residents charts were reviewed retrospectively using the flow sheets. Measures of quality of physician assessment and intervention, quality of nurse assessment and intervention, and global quality were developed and the intra- and interrater reliabilities were tested. The measures' validity was assessed by their ability to predict resident death. Intrarater reliability was measured as the correlation of the ratings of blinded duplicates. Interrater reliability was tested by examining what percentage of the quality ratings were within 1 unit (1 to 5 scale) for all three raters. The subscale of quality of physician assessment was able to predict resident death when the worst episode of care or the mean episode of care was used. None of the other subscales or the global measure predicted death.

Author(s): Kayser-Jones, J.
Article Title: Inadequate staffing at mealtime: Implications for nursing and health policy
Journal Title: *Journal of Gerontological Nursing*
Volume (Issue): 23(8)   **Year:** 1997 (August)   **Pages:** 14–21

Summary: Physicians, nursing staff, residents, and their families concur that staffing is inadequate at mealtimes. Inadequate staffing contributes to residents being fed quickly, forcefully, and sometimes not being fed at all, which results in significant weight loss. To improve mealtime care, it is recommended that (a) nursing homes hire Gerontological Nurse Practitioners or Gerontological Clinical Nurse Specialists to assess residents who are not eating well and develop an individualized care plan for each resident; (b) an RN be on duty 24 hours a day, 7 days a week; (c) each staff member have no more than two to three residents to feed or assist at mealtime; (d) nurses, working with other professionals, take primary responsibility for nutritional care; (e) nursing homes provide a selective menu for residents; and (f) schools of nursing formalize and standardize content in gerontological nursing in their curricula.

Author(s): Kayser-Jones, J., & Schell, E.
Article Title: The mealtime experience of a cognitively impaired elder: Ineffective and effective strategies
Journal Title: *Journal of Gerontological Nursing*
Volume (Issue): 23(7)   **Year:** 1997 (July)   **Pages:** 33–39

Summary: Cognitively impaired residents sometimes exhibit challenging mealtime behaviors that require skillful nursing interventions. Commonly used strategies such as mixing the food together and totally feeding the resident or, conversely, labeling the person uncooperative and providing little supervision and assistance will compromise the resident's dignity and nutritional intake. Strategies that promote independence and that at the same time provide adequate supervision and assistance within a pleasant, social context can enhance nutritional intake and enjoyment of meals.

Author(s): Koroknay, V. J., Werner, P., Cohen-Mansfield, J., & Braun, J. V.
Article Title: Maintaining ambulation in the frail nursing home resident: A nursing administered walking program
Journal Title: *Journal of Gerontological Nursing*
Volume (Issue): 21(11) **Year:** 1995 (November) **Pages:** 18–24

Summary: Because nursing home residents often become dependent on wheelchairs after their admission, a nursing-administered walking program was developed to focus on maintaining mobility in the frail nursing home resident who was in need of assisted ambulation. Nursing assistants played a vital role in ensuring that residents who required assistance with ambulation were in fact ambulated as part of the residents' daily activities. Walking schedules and the goals to be obtained revolve around the nursing unit's activities and the resident's daily activities. Residents who were participants in the walking program experienced an improvement in their ambulatory status and a decrease in falls after participating in the walking program.

Author(s): Kovach, C. R., & Henschel, H.
Article Title: Planning activities for patients with dementia: A descriptive study of therapeutic activities on special care units
Journal Title: *Journal of Gerontological Nursing*
Volume (Issue): 22(9) **Year:** 1996 (September) **Pages:** 33–38

Summary: Therapeutic activities for people with dementia have been used to prevent behavior problems, relieve boredom, and maintain or restore holistic health and function. This study found that subjects spent more time actively participating in an activity when they were able to make a cognitive tie between the current activity and an event from their past through reminiscing. Active participation in therapeutic activities was associated with increased daytime napping but was not related to continuous sleep at night.

Author(s): Kuehn, A. F., & Sendelweck, S.
Article Title: Acute health status and its relationship to falls in the nursing home
Journal Title: *Journal of Gerontological Nursing*
Volume (Issue): 21(7) **Year:** 1995 (July) **Pages:** 41–49

Summary: Falls represent a major health threat to the elderly, often resulting in injury, disability, and/or death. A significant association between acute changes in health status and falling was revealed in this study over 1 month, 2 months, and alternating time periods. Nurses' fall prevention efforts should be more attuned to the more relevant predictor of changing health status and functioning capability of residents.

Author(s): Mylotte, J. M.
Article Title: Measuring antibiotic use in a long-term care facility
Journal Title: *American Journal of Infection Control*
Volume (Issue): 24(3) **Year:** 1996 (June) **Pages:** 174–179

Summary: The objectives of this study were to compare various measures of quantitating antibiotic use and to correlate these measures with febrile morbidity and Foley catheter use in a hospital-based, long-term care facility. This was a prospective study in which the number of residents with fever (rectal temperature of 100.5 °F or greater) or a Foley catheter was documented daily. Between January and December 1989, 111 (71%) of 156 residents were prescribed 263 antibiotic courses. On average, only about 5% of resident care days per month were associated with antibiotic use, whereas an average of 18 residents per month received antibiotic therapy. No significant correlations were found between any antibiotic use measure and febrile days or Foley catheter days each month. In the long-term care facility setting, monitoring the number of residents treated with antibiotics per month is a more practical and useful measure of use than measurement of resident care days on antibiotics per month.

Author(s): Phillips, C. D., Spry, K. M., Sloane, P. D., & Hawes, C.
Article Title: Use of physical restraints and psychotropic medications in Alzheimer special care units in nursing homes
Journal Title: *American Journal of Public Health*
Volume (Issue): 90(1) **Year:** 2000 (January) **Pages:** 92–96

Summary: This study analyzed the use of mechanical restraints and psychotropic medication in Alzheimer special care units (SCUs) in nursing homes. Data from 1993 were analyzed for more than 71,000 nursing home residents in four states, including more than 1100 residents in 48 SCUs. The dependent variable in multinomial logistic regression was use of physical restraints or psychotropic medication. Models contained covariates representing facility and resident characteristics, and multivariate matching strategies were used to protect against selection bias. Residents in SCUs did not differ from similar residents in traditional units in their likelihood of being physically restrained. Residents in SCUs were more likely to receive psychotropic medication. With regard to the measures used in this research, the findings indicate that residents in the SCUs in the four study states did not receive quality of care superior to that provided to similar residents in traditional units. In fact, the results related to drug use raise the question of whether some may have received poorer care.

Author(s): Sheppard, C. M., & Brenner, P. S.
Article Title: The effects of bathing and skin care practices on skin quality and satisfaction with an innovative product
Journal Title: *Journal of Gerontological Nursing*
Volume (Issue): 26(10) **Year:** 2000 (October) **Pages:** 36–45

Summary: Dry skin, the most common skin disorder of the elderly, can be effectively prevented and treated with appropriate bathing and skin care practices. The use of the commercially available Bag Bath/Travel Bath in its design and procedure incorporates many recommendations from the Agency for Health Care Policy and Research (AHCPR) guideline for the prevention of pressure ulcers. The use of the Big Bath/Travel Bath reduced overall skin dryness, more so in the areas of skin flaking and scaling, and less so the areas of redness and cracking. Both residents and nursing staff considered the Bag Bath/Travel Bath an easy, convenient, and effective bathing means that improved skin quality.

Author(s): Simmons, S. F., & Schnelle, J. F.
Article Title: Strategies to measure nursing home residents' satisfaction and preferences related to incontinence and mobility care: Implications for evaluating intervention effects
Journal Title: *The Gerontologist*
Volume (Issue): 39(3) Year: 1999 Pages: 345–355

Summary: This study compared four different interview strategies to measure 111 incontinent nursing home residents' "met need" related to incontinence and mobility care. Strategies were compared on criteria related to ceiling effects and stability. Four methods were used: questions that used the term "satisfaction," direct questions about preferences that did not use the term "satisfaction" that could be translated into three indirect measures of met need. All of these measures were then compared to direct observations of care processes. Residents were more stable in their reports indicating that their care needs were met than they were in their reports that their needs were not met. The direct satisfaction questions produced information most characterized by ceiling effects compared to information elicited by the preference questions. Despite high reported rates of met need as assessed by two of the four methods, direct observations revealed low frequencies of care provision.

Author(s): Stevenson, K. B.
Article Title: Regional data set of infection rates for long-term care facilities: Description of a valuable benchmarking tool
Journal Title: *American Journal of Infection Control*
Volume (Issue): 27(1) Year: 1999 (February) Pages: 20–26

Summary: The aim of this initial study was to create a standardized regional data set of infection rates that could provide an external benchmark for inter-facility comparison. The study included six long-term care facilities in close geographic proximity with similar patient populations. Surveillance in each facility was conducted by a licensed nurse supervised by an infectious diseases physician. Data were pooled in an aggregate cumulative fashion, and data analysis was patterned after the National Nosocomial Infection Surveillance System. The data set consisted of 328,065 resident-days of care during 30 months, with a total of 1252 infections for a pooled mean rate of 3.82 infections per 1000 resident-days of care. Infections for specific categories were 496 urinary tract infections (rate 1.51), 376 respiratory tract infections (rate 1.15), 88 gastroenteritis infections (rate 0.27), 283 skin and soft tissue infections (rate 0.86), 2 bloodstream infections (rate 0.06), and 3 unexplained febrile illnesses (rate 0.09). Data analysis for comparison included interfacility means ± 2 standard deviations and percentiles of distribution. A regional data set of infection rates for long-term care facilities allowed for meaningful interfacility comparison of overall and specific endemic rates and is a valuable benchmarking tool for participating facilities.

Author(s): Van Ort, S., & Phillips, L. R.
Article Title: Nursing interventions to promote functional feeding
Journal Title: *Journal of Gerontological Nursing*
Volume (Issue): 21(10) **Year:** 1995 (October) **Pages:** 7–14

Summary: Results of this study suggest that specific nursing protocols can be designed to promote functional feeding for demented elders in nursing homes while enhancing mealtime environment for both the demented elders and their caregivers. By nurses altering the feeding environment (context) alone, subjects received more food and drink, refused less food, and showed more self-feeding. Major findings were that subjects demonstrated increased independence by refusing food more often and initiating self-feeding more frequently.

Quality Measurement (N = 9)

Author(s): Anderson, R. A., Su, H., Hsieh, P., Allred, C. A., Owensby, S., & Joiner-Rogers, G.
Article Title: Case mix adjustment in nursing systems research: The case of resident outcomes in nursing homes
Journal Title: *Research in Nursing & Health*
Volume (Issue): 22(4) **Year:** 1999 (August) **Pages:** 271–283

Summary: The purpose of this study was to examine selected case mix indicators for their usefulness in separating the variation in outcomes due to differences in resident characteristics versus variation due to differences in nursing care. We explored two methods for combining resident assessment data into a case mix index (CMI). Of the 380 nursing homes contacted, 195 participated, with 164 providing complete data. Two types of case mix indicators were examined in this study. Resident outcomes were defined as the results of nursing care experienced by the residents within each home and were derived from the CARE Form. Ten indicators were selected because they reflected quality of the nursing care. Hierarchical multiple regression analysis was conducted. The prevalence-based, multi-indicator CMI, composed of 22 separate resident risk factors, consistently explained more variance in outcomes than the facility-level, composite CMI. Our findings suggest that the composite CMI does not explain substantial variance in resident outcomes, at least as defined in this study. The inability to discern whether a risk factor was preexisting to an adverse outcome or the result of an adverse outcome increases the potential for overestimating the influence of risk factors on outcomes. Recommendations for further investigation include replicating this study in samples from states that use a different resident assessment form in case mix reimbursement.

Author(s): Bell, P. A., & Smith, J. M.
Article Title: A behavior mapping method for assessing efficacy of change on special care units
Journal Title: *American Journal of Alzheimer's Disease*
Volume (Issue): 12(4) **Year:** 1997 (July–August) **Pages:** 184–189

Summary: A behavior mapping strategy is presented that can be used to quantify the impact of changes in special care units such as new activity programs, increased staff time, or modified floor plans. This article shows how the method was used to compare a newly opened Alzheimer unit with an established Alzheimer unit over a 3-month period. The incidence of clean face and clean clothes at the new unit started out below the frequencies at the established unit, but matched the performance at the established unit by the end of the study. Walking was twice as likely to occur as sleeping during the day. Shouting, swearing, and hitting were extremely rare events. The behavior mapping method could be adapted as one index of quality of care.

Author(s): Hoeffer, B., Rader, J., McKenzie, D., Lavelle, M., & Stewart, B.
Article Title: Reducing aggressive behavior during bathing cognitively impaired nursing home residents
Journal Title: *Journal of Gerontological Nursing*
Volume (Issue): 23(5) **Year:** 1997 (May) **Pages:** 16–23

Summary: Disruptive behaviors, including physical and verbal aggression, often occur during bathing and are especially common among cognitively impaired nursing home residents. The intervention was aimed at changing the psychosocial environment in which bathing occurred and addressed the function, frequency, and form of bathing as well. A model of care that emphasizes an individualized person-focused rather than task-focused approach can reduce aggressive behavior during bathing and make it a more positive caregiving experience for nursing assistants and less distressful for residents.

Author(s): Mukamel, D. B., & Brower, C. A.
Article Title: The influence of risk adjustment methods on conclusions about quality of care in nursing homes based on outcome measures
Journal Title: *Gerontologist*
Volume (Issue): 38(6) **Year:** 1998 (December) **Pages:** 695–703

Summary: This study compares quality rankings of 550 nursing homes in New York state based on several outcome measures and differing risk adjustment methods. The outcomes were decline in functional status, worsening decubiti, and prevalence of physical restraints. Measures were constructed from patient review instrument (PRI) data, which are similar to NMDS data. We found substantial disagreement on quality ranking across measures due to differences in the scope of risk adjustment. Insufficient risk adjustment of outcome measures may, therefore, lead to inappropriate classification of nursing homes as either poor-quality or high-quality homes. This has implications for state quality oversight, providers' reputations, and patients' choice.

Author(s): Pandolph, A., Mazzoni-Maddigan, J., Watzlaf, V. J. M., & Silverman, M.
Article Title: Development of a pilot quality assessment tool for long-term care facilities
Journal Title: *Topics in Health Information Management*
Volume (Issue): 18(1) **Year:** 1997 (August) **Pages:** 23–31

Summary: Recently, the demand to provide exceptional health care services has become of paramount importance. Facilities are competing to provide to the public data that illustrate why one facility is superior to another. One area that has become important is demonstrating the performance of quality of care. The problem with proving the quality of services provided arises from the fact that defining quality as a single entity is difficult. Realizing this factor has created the need to define and measure quality of care in concrete ways. The intent of this research was to facilitate a technique to measure quality of care in long-term care facilities (LTCFs). This research resulted in the development of a pilot quality assessment tool to measure areas of care in LTCFs.

Author(s): Porell, F., & Caro, F. G.
Article Title: Facility-level outcome performance measures for nursing homes
Journal Title: *Gerontologist*
Volume (Issue): 38(6)   **Year:** 1998 (December)   **Pages:** 665–683

Summary: Risk-adjusted nursing home performance scores were developed for four health outcomes and five quality indicators from resident-level longitudinal case-mix reimbursement data for Medicaid residents of more than 500 nursing homes in Massachusetts. Facility performance was measured by comparing actual resident outcomes with expected outcomes derived from quarterly predictions of resident-level econometric models over a 3-year period (1992 to 1994). Performance measures were tightly distributed among facilities in the state. The intercorrelations among the nine outcome performance measures were relatively low and not uniformly positive. Performance measures were not highly associated with various structural facility attributes. For most outcomes, longitudinal analyses revealed only modest correlations between a facility's performance score from one time period to the next. Relatively few facilities exhibited consistently superior or inferior performances over time. The findings have implications for the practical use of facility outcome performance measures for quality assurance and reimbursement purposes in the near future.

Author(s): Rantz, M. J., Mehr, D. R., Popejoy, L., Zwygart-Stauffacher, M., Hicks, L. L., Grando, V., Conn, V. S., Porter, R., Scott, J., & Maas, M.
Article Title: Nursing home care quality: A multidimensional theoretical model
Journal Title: *Journal of Nursing Care Quality*
Volume (Issue): 12(3)   **Year:** 1998 (February)   **Pages:** 30–46, 69–70

Summary: This exploratory study was undertaken to discover the defining dimensions of nursing home care quality and to propose a conceptual model to guide nursing home quality research and the development of instruments to measure nursing home care quality. Three focus groups were conducted in three central Missouri communities. A naturalistic inductive analysis of the transcribed content was completed. Two core variables (interaction and odor) and several related concepts emerged from the data. The seven dimensions of the multidimensional model of nursing home care quality are central focus, interaction, milieu, environment, individualized care, staff, and safety. To pursue quality, the many dimensions must be of primary concern to nursing homes. We are testing an instrument based on the model to observe and score the dimensions of nursing home care quality.

Author(s): Rantz, M. J., Zwygart-Stauffacher, M., Popejoy, L., Grando, V. T., Mehr, D. R., Hicks, L. L., Conn, V. S., Wipke-Tevis, D., Porter, R., Bostick, J., & Maas, M.
Article Title: Nursing home care quality: A multidimensional theoretical model integrating the views of consumers and providers
Journal Title: *Journal of Nursing Care Quality*
Volume (Issue): 14(1)   **Year:** 1999 (October)   **Pages:** 16–37, 85–87

Summary: This exploratory study was undertaken to discover the defining dimensions of nursing home care quality from the viewpoint of consumers of nursing home care. Eleven focus groups were conducted in five Missouri communities. The seven dimensions of the consumer multidimensional model of nursing home care quality are staff, care, family involvement, communication, environment, home, and cost. The views of consumers and families are compared with the results of a previous study of providers of nursing home services. An integrated, multidimensional theoretical model is presented for testing and evaluation. An instrument based on the model is being tested to observe and score the dimensions of nursing home care quality.

Author(s): Rantz, M. J., Mehr, D. R., Petroski, G. F., Madsen, R. W., Popejoy, L. L., Hicks, L. L., Conn, V. S., Grando, V. T., Wipke-Tevis, D. D., Bostick, J., Porter, R., Zwygart-Stauffacher, M., & Maas, M.
Article Title: Initial field testing of an instrument to measure: Observable indicators of nursing home care quality
Journal Title: *Journal of Nursing Care Quality*
Volume (Issue): 14(3)   **Year:** 2000 (April)   **Pages:** 1–12

Summary: The "Observable Indicators of Nursing Home Care Quality" instrument was developed as a new measure of nursing home care quality. The instrument is based on a theoretical model of quality nursing home care grounded in data from provider and consumer focus groups. The instrument was tested in 10 Missouri nursing homes. Subsequent versions were tested in 109 Missouri and 11 Icelandic nursing homes. Content validity was established using experts. Concurrent and known groups validity was evaluated using NMDS quality indicators, survey citations, and a process of care measure. Interrater and test–retest reliabilities were calculated as well as coefficient alpha. The "Observable Indicators of Nursing Home Care Quality" instrument is a new measure that can be used by researchers, and potentially by regulators, consumers, or providers, to observe and score specific indicators of quality care following a 20- to 30-minute inspection of a nursing home.

Staffing (N = 8)

Author(s): Anderson, R. A., & McDaniel, R. R. Jr.
Article Title: RN participation in organizational decision making and improvements in resident outcomes
Journal Title: *Health Care Management Review*
Volume (Issue): 24(1)   **Year:** 1999 (Winter)   **Pages:** 7–16

Summary: In the study on which this article is based, nursing homes with the most improvements in resident outcomes had greater registered nurse (RN) participation in decision making than did homes with the least improvements. The results suggest that nursing homes that want to improve quality can use RN participation to make improvements without significantly increasing costs. Complexity theory served as a framework for the study.

Author(s): Anderson, R. A., Hsieh, P., & Su, H.
Article Title: Resource allocation and resident outcomes in nursing homes: Comparisons between the best and worst
Journal Title: *Research in Nursing & Health*
Volume (Issue): 21(4)   **Year:** 1998 (August)   **Pages:** 297–313

Summary: The purpose of this study was to identify patterns of resource allocation that relate to resident outcomes in nursing homes. Secondary data were obtained from the Texas Department of Human Services (TDHS) for all nursing homes in the state. Data on staffing levels and financial resources were obtained from the 1990 Medicaid Nursing Facility Cost Reports and data on case mix and resident outcomes were obtained from the 1990 Client Assessment, Reviews, and Evaluation Form. The group with the best outcomes were larger, had more non-profit homes, and a greater percentage of private pay residents. The greatest improvement in resident outcomes was found in smaller, for-profit homes. Raw means show that the group with the best average outcomes had more RN full-time employees per 60 beds and a greater percentage of RNs in the staff mix. The group of nursing homes with the greatest improvement in resident outcomes provided more RN staffing and spent more per day than the group with the least improvement. The results suggest two main conclusions: (a) improvements in resident outcomes requires RN staffing; and (b) because of the need for RN staffing, improvements in resident outcomes requires greater spending.

Author(s): Bowers, B. J., Esmond, S., & Jacobson, N.
Article Title: The relationship between staffing and quality in long-term care facilities: Exploring the views of nurse aides
Journal Title: *Journal of Nursing Care Quality*
Volume (Issue): 14(4)   **Year:** 2000 (July)   **Pages:** 55–64, 73–75

Summary: Research on staffing and quality of care in LTCFs confirms that adequate staffing levels are important to ensuring quality, but few studies have examined how the two are linked. The research reported in this article used participant observation and in-depth interviewing to explore how nurse aides understand the link between staffing and quality. The findings show that nurses aides deem their relationships with residents to be the central determinant of quality of care as well as an important outcome in itself. Adequate staffing is essential to allowing nurses aides to nurture these relationships.

Author(s): Harrington, C., Zimmerman, D., Karon, S. L., Robinson, J., & Beutel, P.
Article Title: Nursing home staffing and its relationship to deficiencies
Journal Title: *Journals of Gerontology Series B—Psychological Sciences & Social Sciences*
Volume (Issue): 55B(5)   **Year:** 2000 (September)   **Pages:** S278–S287

Summary: The authors examined the relationships between different types of nursing home staffing and nursing home deficiencies to test the hypothesis that fewer staff hours would be associated with higher numbers of deficiencies. Data were from the On-Line Survey, Certification, and Reporting System for all certified nursing homes in the United States. Regression models examined total deficiencies, quality of care, quality of life, and other deficiencies. Fewer registered nurse hours and nursing assistant hours were associated with total deficiencies and quality of care deficiencies when other variables were controlled. Fewer nursing assistant staff and other care staff hours were associated with quality of life deficiencies. Fewer administrative staff hours were associated with other deficiencies. Facilities that had more depressed and demented residents, that were smaller, and that were nonprofit or government-owned had fewer deficiencies. Facilities with more residents with urinary incontinence and pressure sores and with higher percentages of Medicaid residents had more deficiencies when staffing and resident characteristics were controlled. Facility characteristics and states were stronger predictors of deficiencies than were staffing hours and resident characteristics.

Author(s): Johnson-Pawlson, J., & Infeld, D. L.
Article Title: Nurse staffing and quality of care in nursing facilities
Journal Title: *Journal of Gerontological Nursing*
Volume (Issue): 22(8)   **Year:** 1996 (August)   **Pages:** 36–45

Summary: Findings of this study indicate that there is a relationship between the ratio of total nursing staff to residents and quality of care as measured by nursing-related nursing home deficiencies. Staffing at higher than federally required minimum levels present cost-quality tradeoffs. Lack of a relationship between the ratio of RNs to residents and quality of care may reflect the limited number of RNs working in nursing facilities.

Author(s): Schirm, V., Albanese, T., Garland, T. N., Gipson, G., & Blackmon, D. J.
Article Title: Caregiving in nursing homes: Views of licensed nurses and nursing assistants
Journal Title: *Clinical Nursing Research*
Volume (Issue): 9(3)   **Year:** 2000 (August)   **Pages:** 280–297

Summary: This investigation is a qualitative study of the views held by 36 licensed nurses (25 RNs and 11 licensed practical nurses) and 40 nursing assistants regarding caregiving in nursing homes. Because these care providers are most directly involved in the delivery of care, their views are important as determinants of quality of care. Study findings focus on the extent to which nurses and nursing assistants agree on what contributes to good care and how they perceive the work that each does. Also reported are their perceptions regarding factors that make care delivery easy or difficult. Results suggest that nurses and nursing assistants share selected perceptions about the division of labor in the nursing home. Also evident are areas of less agreement among these members of different status sets. A discussion of how these caregivers can work together as effective team members is presented.

Author(s): Schirm, V., Albanese, T., & Garland, T. N.
Article Title: Understanding nursing home quality of care: Incorporating caregivers' perceptions through structure, process, and outcome
Journal Title: *Quality Management in Health Care*
Volume (Issue): 8(1)   **Year:** 1999 (Fall)   **Pages:** 55–63

Summary: This article describes a study that was developed in response to the increasing work in humanistic or healing environment models and the need for validation of the advantages of such models. A descriptive correlational survey design was applied to explore relationships between overall job satisfaction and staff ($N = 192$) perceptions of the extent to which the healing model incorporates (1) common understandings of health as a function of body-mind-spirit interrelationships, (2) patient-centered relationships that are caring focused, and (3) a culture supportive of personal growth and mastery within the setting of Yavapai Regional Medical Center, a 100-bed facility in rural Arizona known for its established healing environment. Case study time-series analysis methods were also used to examine trends in organizational performance and comparison of performance to regional norms. The healthy organization model, a framework for health care organizations that incorporates humanistic healing values within the traditional structure, was presented as a result of the study. This model addresses the importance of optimal clinical services, financial performance, and staff satisfaction.

Author(s): Singh, D. A., Amidon, R. L., Shi, L., & Samuels, M. E.
Article Title: Predictors of quality of care in nursing facilities
Journal Title: *Journal of Long Term Care Administration*
Volume (Issue): 24(3)   **Year:** 1996 (Fall)   **Pages:** 22–26

Summary: Administrators with nursing backgrounds, who spend time in patient care management and who have long tenure have strong positive influence on their facilities' quality of care.

MDS/Quality Indicators (N = 8)

Author(s): Arling, G., Karon, S. L., Sainfort, F., Zimmerman, D. R., & Ross, R.
Article Title: Risk adjustment of nursing home quality indicators
Journal Title: *Gerontologist*
Volume (Issue): 37(6)   **Year:** 1997 (December)   **Pages:** 757–766

Summary: The purpose of this study was to develop a method for risk adjusting nursing home quality indicators (QIs). The QIs measure incidence and prevalence of resident-level care processes and outcomes that are indicative of care quality. Risk adjustment was carried out by stratifying residents into risk groups (high and low), calculating QI rates within groups, and then drawing comparisons across facilities. The method was examined through analysis of data from over 800 nursing homes in four states. Results showed that facilities differed substantially in QI rates even after risk had been taken into account. Also, results suggested differences in care quality that may not have been apparent without controlling for risk.

Author(s): Marek, K. D., Rantz, M. J., Fagin, C. M., & Krejci, J. W.
Article Title: OBRA '87: Has it resulted in better quality of care?
Journal Title: *Journal of Gerontological Nursing*
Volume (Issue): 22(10) Year: 1996 (October) Pages: 28–36

Summary: Post-OBRA implementation, the focus of care has shifted from provider-driven to resident-driven. The NMDS is a useful tool providing a more comprehensive perspective of patient care. Implementation of PASARR has been problematic and should be examined.

Author(s): Mentes, J., Culp, K., Maas, M., & Rantz, M.
Article Title: Acute confusion indicators: Risk factors and prevalence using MDS data
Journal Title: *Research in Nursing & Health*
Volume (Issue): 22(2) Year: 1999 (April) Pages: 95–105

Summary: The purpose of this cross-sectional study was to use NMDS data to test whether risk variables derived from a conceptual model predicted acute confusion in long-term care residents. The sample was composed predominantly of women ($n = 1775$). Based on the conceptual model and items available in the NMDS, precipitating factors selected for analysis were dehydration, hypoxia, infections, and medications. Frequencies of the indicators suggest that cognitive ability variation and periods of motor restlessness/ lethargy are the most readily recognized symptoms of acute confusion by nursing home staff. The only variables that contributed to the explanation of acute confusion in the logistic regression analysis were inadequate fluid intake, dementia status, and a fall in the past 30 days. The strongest contributing factor to acute confusion in this population was inadequate fluid intake. Although medications are the most frequent cause of acute confusion in older hospital patients, this was not the case in these LTCF residents.

Author(s): Phillips, C. D., Zimmerman, D., Bernabei, R., & Jonsson, P. V.
Article Title: Using the Resident Assessment Instrument for quality enhancement in nursing homes
Journal Title: *Age & Ageing*
Volume (Issue): 26(Suppl 2) Year: 1997 Pages: 77–81

Summary: In some current policy discussions concerning long-term care, the emphasis has been almost solely on the costs of care. This dialogue must be replaced with a discussion of value, which emphasizes both the costs of care and quality of care. Although the Resident Assessment Instrument (RAI) was originally designed as a multidimensional assessment tool aimed at improving clinical practice, it can also provide the foundation for a comprehensive data base that can be used to assess and monitor the quality of care. Using data from four sites (in Denmark, Iceland, Italy and the United States) and eight indicators of quality that could be derived from single assessments, the authors demonstrate how quality might be measured and compared using the RAI. Although this is for illustrative purposes only, it does show how this database can provide invaluable information to providers about the quality of care within their facilities. It can also allow consumers and purchasers to evaluate the relative performance of different providers.

Author(s): Rantz, M. J., Mehr, D. R., Conn, V. S., Hicks, L. L., Porter, R., Madsen, R. W., Petroski, G. F., & Maas, M.
Article Title: Assessing quality of nursing home care: The foundation for improving resident outcomes
Journal Title: *Journal of Nursing Care Quality*
Volume (Issue): 10(4)   **Year:** 1996 (July)   **Pages:** 1–9

Summary: The article describes a study that analyzed the QIs identified by the Health Care Financing Administration (HCFA)-sponsored Case Mix and Quality Demonstration Project using the Missouri nursing home NMDS database. The range of performance was considerable, and five of the indicators analyzed were risk adjusted to account for variation in resident acuity within facilities. Determining quality of care from assessment information that is routinely collected for nursing home residents has the potential to dramatically influence public policy decisions regarding reimbursement, recertification, and regulation and can play a vital role in improving resident outcomes.

Author(s): Rantz, M. J., Popejoy, L., Mehr, D. R., Zwygart-Stauffacher, M., Hicks, L. L., Grando, V., Conn, V. S., Porter, R., Scott, J., & Maas, M.
Article Title: Verifying nursing home care quality using Minimum Data Set quality indicators and other quality measures
Journal Title: *Journal of Nursing Care Quality*
Volume (Issue): 12(2)   **Year:** 1997 (December)   **Pages:** 54–62

Summary: Researchers, providers, and government agencies have devoted time and resources to the development of a set of QIs derived from NMDS data. Little effort has been directed toward verifying that QIs derived from NMDS data accurately measure nursing home quality. Researchers at the University of Missouri—Columbia have independently verified the accuracy of QI derived from NMDS data using four different methods: (1) structured participative observation, (2) QI Observation Scoring Instrument, (3) Independent Observable Indicators of Quality Instrument, and (4) survey citations. The authors were able to determine that QIs derived from NMDS data did differentiate nursing homes of good quality from those of poorer quality.

Author(s): Rantz, M. J., Petroski, G. F., Madsen, R. W., Scott, J., Mehr, D. R., Popejoy, L., Hicks, L. L., Porter, R., Zwygart-Stauffacher, M., & Grando, V. T.
Article Title: Setting thresholds for MDS quality indicators for nursing home quality improvement reports
Journal Title: *Journal of Quality Improvement*
Volume (Issue): 23(11)   **Year:** 1997   **Pages:** 602–611

Summary: The NMDS assessment instrument is mandated for use nationwide in all nursing homes participating in Medicaid or Medicare programs. In July 1996, a cross-section of 13 clinical care personnel from nursing homes participated on an expert panel for threshold setting for QIs derived from NMDS assessment data. Panel members individually determined good and poor threshold scores for each QI, reviewed statewide distributions of NMDS QIs and, 2 weeks later completed a follow-up Delphi round. Three members of the research team reviewed the results of the expert panel and set the final thresholds. With thresholds established for good and poor scores, NMDS QI scores are reported to a sample of Missouri nursing homes using the thresholds. To ensure that thresholds reflect current practice, threshold setting with another panel of experts will be repeated as needed, but at least biannually. The report format will be revised on the basis of user input, and a statewide study testing different educational support methods for quality improvement using NMDS QIs is underway.

Author(s): Rantz, M. J., Petroski, G. F., Madsen, R. W., Mehr, D. R., Popejoy, L., Hicks, L. L., Porter, R., Zwygart-Stauffacher, M., & Grando, V.
Article Title: Setting thresholds for quality indicators derived from MDS data for nursing home quality improvement reports: An update
Journal Title: *Journal on Quality Improvement*
Volume (Issue): 26(2)   **Year:** 2000   **Pages:** 101–110

Summary: This article builds on the work of an earlier panel of experts that set thresholds for QIs derived from the NMDS assessment data. Thresholds were now set for the revised MDS 2.0 two-page quarterly form Resource Utilization Groups III (RUGS III) quarterly instrument. Panel members individually determined lower (good) and upper (poor) threshold scores for each QI, reviewed statewide distributions of NMDS QIs, and completed a follow-up Delphi of the final results. The QI reports compiled longitudinal data for all residents in the nursing home during each quarter and cumulatively displayed data for five quarters for each QI. Quality improvement teams found the reports helpful and easy to interpret. As the NMDS instrument or recommended calculations for the NMDS QIs change, thresholds will be reestablished to ensure a fit with the instrument and data.

Satisfaction with Care (N = 5)

Author(s): Heliker, D. M.
Article Title: A narrative approach to quality care in long-term care facilities
Journal Title: *Journal of Holistic Nursing*
Volume (Issue): 15(1)   **Year:** 1997 (March)   **Pages:** 68–81

Summary: The negative effects of institutionalization caused partially by homogeneity and uniformity of care prompts the exploration of personal and common meanings of nursing home residents. This study is viewed as an initial step in providing quality care as defined by the resident. Personal and common meanings embedded in the lived lives of five older women residing in a LTCF are interpreted using a seven-stage Heideggerian hermeneutical phenomenological approach. An unstructured modified life review format is used to interview each participant on three separate occasions. Three constitutive patterns emerge: dwelling in remembering, living relatedly, and being after loss. These patterns endure across the lifespan of each woman and continue to endure after admission to the facility. The revelation of common and personal meanings provides new possibilities for the transformation of nursing practice to ensure quality care from the perspective of what is considered meaningful to each resident.

Author(s): Meister, C., & Boyle, C.
Article Title: Perceptions of quality in long-term care: A satisfaction survey
Journal Title: *Journal of Nursing Care Quality*
Volume (Issue): 10(4) **Year:** 1996 (July) **Pages:** 40–47

Summary: At a 387-bed geriatric hospital in Montreal, Canada, a cross-sectional satisfaction survey was conducted on random samples of patients, families, families of deceased patients, and nursing staff. Using the same pretested structured questionnaire, the subjects were asked to rank (assign importance to) and rate (assign a rate of success to) 15 indicators of quality care. Significant differences both between and within the four groups were found on the perceived importance and rate of success of many of the indicators, supporting the primary hypotheses. Ethnicity and several sociodemographic covariates influenced the importance and rate of success assigned to the key indicators. The article discusses survey methodology issues as well as the integration of a satisfaction survey into an overall quality improvement program.

Author(s): Steffen, T. M., & Nystrom, P. C.
Article Title: Validation of a measure of family members' perceptions of service quality in nursing homes
Journal Title: *Journal of Rehabilitation Outcomes Measurement*
Volume (Issue): 1(4) **Year:** 1997 (August) **Pages:** 1–9

Summary: This field study examined primary data collected from over 350 family members of persons living in 41 skilled nursing facilities. Twenty-one question from the SERVQUAL questionnaire measured the quality dimensions of Responsiveness, Reliability, Assurance, Empathy, and Tangibles. Results corroborate the reliability and validity of this service quality measure for use in nursing homes. SERVQUAL is an easy-to-administer measure of family members' satisfaction with service quality in nursing homes.

Author(s): Wakefield, B., Buckwalter, K. C., & Collins, C. E.
Article Title: Assessing family satisfaction with care for persons with dementia
Journal Title: *Balance*
Volume (Issue): 1(1) **Year:** 1997 (July) **Pages:** 16–17, 40–42

Summary: The data for this study were collected as a part of a national survey of SCUs, supported by the Alzheimer's Association. The family questionnaire surveyed demographics, facility data, and the families' experience with care in Alzheimer's SCUs. Overall family perceptions of SCUs were equal to or better than group homes, whereas nursing homes scored consistently lower on these ratings. Group homes and nursing homes scored about the same on variables related to admission and care practices. Higher satisfaction in SCUs may reflect the greater importance placed on family involvement in these units.

Author(s): Watson, C. J., Mobarak, A. M., & Stimson, K.
Article Title: A collaborative effort to establish a long-term care benchmark process
Journal Title: *Journal for Healthcare Quality*
Volume (Issue): 21(2)   Year: 1999   Pages: 19–23

Summary: This article describes a benchmark process, developed and implemented in a not-for profit LTCF in the Rochester, New York area. A resident expectation survey was developed, which examined 44 aspects of care or service. A resident satisfaction survey was also developed and administered to residents ($n = 121$) in nine participating facilities. Based on analysis of resident surveys, it was determined that the issue of missing clothing would be benchmarked. Data relationships detailing desired outcomes were identified as: the number of items lost in relation to total production, the number of items recovered in relation to items reported lost, and the number of items recovered within 7 days in relation to total items recovered. Implementation of the benchmark process resulted in an increase in clothing recovery rate from 37 to 75% in the first month. This facility continued to be successful having an 84% recovery rate in 1997, with 87% of the items recovered within 7 days.

Family Involvement (N = 2)

Author(s): Friedemann, M., Montgomery, R. J., Maiberger, B., & Smith, A. A.
Article Title: Family involvement in the nursing home: Family-oriented practices and staff-family relations
Journal Title: *Research in Nursing & Health*
Volume (Issue): 20(6)   Year: 1997 (December)   Pages: 527–537

Summary: The purpose of this study was to investigate family involvement patterns, staff–family interactions, and nursing home factors that families perceive as helpful or inhibiting. Twenty-four homes were selected at random. All family members of residents admitted to these 24 homes over a 22-month period were invited to a telephone interview. The interview data were analyzed using a qualitative approach to content analysis. Problems were cited by 63% of families, and each family described an average of 2.7 problems. Frequently, resident care problems concerned the dignity (identity) of the patient in that staff did not view residents as persons with rights. Family interaction problems were cited more frequently than any others. In spite of the large number of problems cited, family members pointed out the many strengths of the staff and the nursing home. The nursing home policies and practices meant to encourage family involvement were found to be, at least to some degree, congruent with the families' actual involvement. The nursing home survey and qualitative data from the families indicated that there were family-oriented homes that promoted learning and gave the families opportunities to be heard and be part of their operation.

Author(s): Specht, J. P., Kelley, L. S., Manion, P., Maas, M. L., Reed, D., & Rantz, M. R.
Article Title: Who's the boss? Family/staff partnership in care of persons with dementia
Journal Title: *Nursing Administration Quarterly*
Volume (Issue): 24(3)   **Year:** 2000 (Spring)   **Pages:** 64–75

Summary: This article provides an overview of family involvement in care intervention and its implementation with African-American and Caucasian family members of persons with dementia in nursing home settings. On the measure of family satisfaction with care, African-American family caregivers were significantly less satisfied than Caucasian family caregivers. The Caucasian family members were generally less satisfied with activities.

End of Life (N = 2)

Author(s): Baer, W. M., & Hanson, L. C.
Article Title: Families' perception of the added value of hospice in the nursing home
Journal Title: *Journal of the American Geriatrics Society*
Volume (Issue): 48(8)   **Year:** 2000 (August)   **Pages:** 879–882

Summary: The purpose of this study was to determine if family members perceive that hospice improves the care of dying nursing home residents during the last 3 months of life. Mailed surveys were sent to family members for all nursing home hospice enrollees in North Carolina during a 6-month period. After residents' deaths, family members answered questions about the quality of care for symptoms before and after hospice, the added value of hospice, the effect of hospice on hospitalization, and special services provided by nursing home staff or by hospice staff. A total of 292 (73%) of 398 eligible family members completed surveys. Quality of care for physical symptoms was rated good or excellent by 64% of family before hospice and 93% after hospice. Dying residents' emotional needs included care for moderate or severe depression (47%), anxiety (50%), and loneliness (35%). Quality of care for emotional needs was rated good or excellent by 64% of family before hospice and 90% after hospice. Fifty-three percent of respondents believed hospice prevented hospitalizations. Family estimated the median added value of hospice to be $75 per day and described distinct special services provided by hospice and by nursing home staff. Family members believe that nursing home hospice improves quality of care for symptoms, reduces hospitalizations, and adds value and services for dying nursing home residents.

Author(s): Tolle, S. W., Tilden, V. P., Nelson, C. A., & Dunn, P. M.
Article Title: A prospective study of the efficacy of the physician order form for life-sustaining treatment
Journal Title: *Journal of the American Geriatrics Society*
Volume (Issue): 46(9)   **Year:** 1998 (September)   **Pages:** 1097–1102

Summary: The Physician Orders for Life-Sustaining Treatment (POLST), a comprehensive, one-page order form, was developed to convey preferences for life-sustaining treatments during transfer from one care site to another. This study examined the extent to which the POLST form ensured that nursing home residents' wishes were honored for do not resuscitate (DNR) and requests for transfer only if comfort measures fail. Nursing home residents (*n* = 180) who had a POLST recording DNR designation and who indicated a desire for transfer only if comfort measures failed, were followed for 1 year. No study subject received CPR, ICU care, or ventilator support, and only 2% were hospitalized to extend life. Of the 38 subjects who died during the study year, 63% had an order for narcotics, and only two (5%) died in an acute care hospital. A total of 24 subjects (13%) were hospitalized during the year. In 85% of all hospitalizations, patients were transferred because the nursing home could not control suffering. In 15% of hospitalizations (*n* = 4), the transfer was to extend life, overriding POLST orders. POLST orders regarding CPR in nursing home residents in this study were universally respected. Study subjects received remarkably high levels of comfort care and low rates of transfer for aggressive life-extending treatments.

Nursing Quality Measurement Studies That Cross All Settings | 8

Overview

The articles in this chapter describe clinical or measurement issues across health care settings that were not limited to one site. The majority of studies dealt with quality improvement initiatives in an integrated health care delivery, managed care, or statewide system. A major challenge identified within these studies is that documentation is often inconsistent across different sites of care. This demonstrates the need for standardized language and a classification system that identifies appropriate outcomes for patients in different settings. Future research is needed to determine what constitutes appropriate outcomes for patients in different settings.

The 18 nursing quality measurement studies in this chapter are organized as follows:

- Quality improvement
- Clinical issues
- Managed care
- Satisfaction with care

Quality Improvement (N = 6)

Author(s): Castaneda-Mendez, K., Mangan, K., & Lavery, A. M.
Article Title: The role and application of the balanced scorecard in healthcare quality management
Journal Title: *Journal for Healthcare Quality*
Volume (Issue): 20(1) **Year:** 1998 **Pages:** 10–13

Summary: To connect practices, outcomes, quality, value, and costs, health care organizations must start using a balanced scorecard. A balanced scorecard is a set of measures that reveal the interdependency of the organization, its employees, and its patients. It thus serves as a balanced perspective on the organization for senior management to use in designing, developing, deploying, and directing the strategic plan, consistent with total quality management (TQM) principles.

Author(s): Green, P. L.
Article Title: Improving clinical effectiveness in an integrated care delivery system
Journal Title: *Journal for Healthcare Quality*
Volume (Issue): 20(6)   Year: 1998   Pages: 4–8

Summary: This article describes the development, implementation, and evaluation of a multidisciplinary care management program in an integrated care delivery system based in St. Paul, Minnesota. The three major components of care management identified were (1) use of tools such as pathways, standing orders, decision algorithms, and patient education materials, (2) establishment of care management teams, and (3) establishment of "collaborative practice committees." Each team identified critical data to be monitored and developed individual measurement plans. A number of program achievements are reported for 1993 through 1996.

Author(s): Jennings, B. M., & Staggers, N.
Article Title: A provocative look at performance measurement
Journal Title: *Nursing Administration Quarterly*
Volume (Issue): 24(1)   Year: 1999 (Fall)   Pages: 17–30

Summary: A fascinating web of issues can be spun from the notion of performance measurement. After a brief discussion about the background of performance measurement, this article puts performance measurement into a fresh light by examining three major issues: the concept of quality and its application to performance measurement, the power of the patient and the transition of focus to customers within health care organizations, and deliberations about data and concomitant implications for information systems of the future.

Author(s): Kroll, D. A., Brummitt, C. F., & Berry, B. B.
Article Title: A users group approach to quality improvement across an integrated healthcare delivery system
Journal Title: *Journal for Healthcare Quality*
Volume (Issue): 22(1)   Year: 2000   Pages: 39–43

Summary: This article describes the Users Group approach to quality improvement (QI) at Aurora Healthcare in southeastern Wisconsin. Only 71% of patients received timely preoperative antibiotic prophylaxis in five Aurora hospitals prior to the QI initiative. A Users Group approach was proposed to foster collaboration among the hospitals. Although these hospitals differed in size, volume of cases, medical staff, and antibiotic-delivery processes, they had common objectives and, many times, common barriers to the timely delivery of antibiotics. The QI effort resulted in an 18% improvement in the number of patients who received timely administration of preoperative antibiotic prophylaxis.

Author(s): Oermann, M. H., & Wilson, F. L.
Article Title: Quality of care information for consumers on the Internet
Journal Title: *Journal of Nursing Care Quality*
Volume (Issue): 14(4)   **Year:** 2000 (July)   **Pages:** 45–54

Summary: The purpose of this study was to assess the readability of quality of care information for consumers available on the Internet. Ten Internet resources for consumers, found at three major web sites, were analyzed for readability. The scores ranged from a low of 6th grade level for information in the document "Quick Checks for Quality: Choosing Quality Health Care" to a high of 12th grade level for "Helping You Choose a Quality Ambulatory Care Organization." The overall mean reading demands of four of the documents were higher than the 8th grade level recommended for the general public. Six of the documents were at this level or below, placing them at an appropriate reading level for most consumers to understand the information.

Author(s): Sloss, E. M., Solomon, D. H., Shekelle, P. G., Young, R. T., Saliba, D., MacLean, C. H., Rubenstein, L. Z., Schnelle, J. F., Kamberg, C. J., & Wenger, N. S.
Article Title: Selecting target conditions for quality of care improvement in vulnerable older adults
Journal Title: *Journal of the American Geriatrics Society*
Volume (Issue): 48(4)   **Year:** 2000 (April)   **Pages:** 363–369

Summary: The purpose of this study was to identify a set of geriatric conditions as optimal targets for quality improvement to be used in a quality measurement system for vulnerable older adults. A panel of 12 experts in geriatric care selected 21 conditions as targets for quality improvement among vulnerable older adults. They include (in rank order) pharmacologic management, depression; dementia, heart failure, stroke (and atrial fibrillation), hospitalization and surgery, falls and mobility disorders, diabetes mellitus, end-of-life care, ischemic heart disease, hypertension, pressure ulcers, osteoporosis, urinary incontinence, pain management, preventive services, hearing impairment, pneumonia and influenza, vision impairment, malnutrition, and osteoarthritis. The 21 target conditions account for at least 43% of all acute hospital discharges and 33% of physician office visits among persons 65 years of age and older. Actual figures must be higher because several of the selected conditions (eg, end-of-life care) are not recorded as diagnoses. The 21 geriatric conditions selected are highly prevalent in this group and likely account for more than half of the care provided to this group in hospital and ambulatory settings.

Clinical Issues (N = 6)

Author(s): Agins, B., Young, M., Ellis, W., Burke, G., & Rotunno, F.
Article Title: A statewide program to evaluate the quality of care provided to persons with HIV infection
Journal Title: *The Joint Commission Journal on Quality Improvement*
Volume (Issue): 21(9)   **Year:** 1995   **Pages:** 439–456

Summary: The purpose of this study was to develop a state-based system for evaluating the quality of HIV clinical services in one state using techniques of continuous quality improvement (CQI). Data compiled from quality of care reviews were grouped according to facility type. Comparative results based on 1575 records in year one and 1829 records in year two presented by facility type indicated consistent performance in HIV disease staging, PCP prophylaxis, and antiretroviral therapy, as well as improvement in performance of pelvic examination. This HIV-specific quality of care evaluation program shows that regulatory bodies can depart from traditional review techniques and adopt more effective and positive means of improving care. This program can serve as a model for developing government-sponsored, CQI-based quality monitoring programs for use with other chronic illnesses and in diverse clinical settings.

Author(s): Forbes, S. A., Duncan, P. W., & Zimmerman, M. K.
Article Title: Review criteria for stroke rehabilitation outcomes
Journal Title: *Archives of Physical Medicine & Rehabilitation*
Volume (Issue): 78(10) **Year:** 1997 (October) **Pages:** 1112–1116

Summary: A descriptive cross-sectional study using a convenience sample was conducted to develop review criteria from the Agency for Health Care Policy and Research (AHCPR) Stroke Rehabilitation Guidelines. Review criteria, developed directly from the AHCPR Stroke Rehabilitation guidelines, consisted of 11 global quality criteria representative of comprehensive multidisciplinary rehabilitative care. There were approximately 150 variables, comprised of specific criteria to measure each of the 11 global quality criteria plus comprehensive demographic and client-specific information. Results of this study suggest that differences exist in documentation of care across the three sites of care. Based on chart documentation, there is variability in the process of stroke rehabilitation care across nursing facilities, inpatient rehabilitation facilities, and home health care. This study provides the impetus for future research specifically evaluating the associations between documentation of the processes of care and patient outcomes.

Author(s): Jones, M. E., & Bond, M. L.
Article Title: Predictors of birth outcome among Hispanic immigrant women
Journal Title: *Journal of Nursing Care Quality*
Volume (Issue): 14(1) **Year:** 1999 (October) **Pages:** 56–62

Summary: This article reports on maternal acculturation status and the relationship to birth outcomes of 382 Hispanic pregnant women in the southwest United States. The majority of these women were Mexican-oriented and had healthy pregnancies and healthy birth outcomes. Findings support the hypothesis that traditional Mexican cultural practices serve protective functions for the childbearing woman.

Author(s): Lynne, J., Schall, M. W., Milne, C., Nolan, K. M., & Kabcenell, A.
Article Title: Quality improvements in end of life care: Insights from two collaboratives

Journal Title: *Journal on Quality Improvement*
Volume (Issue): 26(5) **Year:** 2000 **Pages:** 254–267

Summary: People usually die from serious chronic disease after a substantial period of disability. Current care systems do not serve this population well. This study looked at two quality improvement collaboratives sponsored by the Institute for Healthcare Improvement and the Center to Improve Care of the Dying, which set about making substantial improvements.

Author(s): Shindul-Rothschild, J., Berry, D., & Long-Middleton, E.,
Article Title: Where have all the nurses gone? Final results of AJN's patient care survey
Journal Title: *MCN, American Journal of Maternal Child Nursing*
Volume (Issue): 22(1) **Year:** 1997 (January–February) **Pages:** 33–47

Summary: We all know the changes in our health care system have been substantial and far-reaching, but what affects are downsizing, restructuring, and the use of unlicensed personnel having on the quality of patient care you deliver and on your work life? More than 7000 survey respondents gave their answers.

Author(s): Zwygart-Stauffacher, M., Lindquist, R., & Savik, K.
Article Title: Development of health care delivery systems that are sensitive to the needs of stroke survivors and their caregivers
Journal Title: *Nursing Administration Quarterly*
Volume (Issue): 24(3) **Year:** 2000 (Spring) **Pages:** 33–42

Summary: The life-altering event of a stroke has long-term effects not only on stroke survivors but also on their caregivers, health care professionals, and health care delivery systems. The nurse-administrator is faced with an obvious challenge to organize nursing systems to meet the multiple needs of the stroke survivor. The article presents data on the perceived needs of stroke survivors and their caregivers that provide direction and assistance to nursing administrators in organizing nursing services to address these perceived needs.

Managed Care (N = 4)

Author(s): Ellenbecker, C. H., Wagner, L., & Cloutterbuck, J.
Article Title: Using insurance claims data and medical record reviews to assess the quality of medical care
Journal Title: *Journal for Healthcare Quality*
Volume (Issue): 19(3) **Year:** 1997 **Pages:** 21–31

Summary: This article examines the possibilities and limitations of using computerized insurance claims and outpatient medical records to evaluate a Medicaid managed care program. The quality of medical care delivered to enrollees 1½ years into the MassHealth managed care program's operation is discussed in the context of an evaluation that was conducted by the University of Massachusetts—Boston's McCormack Institute in 1993. Study results suggest that these two data sources offer adequate information to determine the quality level of primary and preventive services and lead to further suggestions for evaluating care.

Author(s): Ipsen, S. K., Fosbinder, D., Williams, M., Warnick, M., Lertwachara, K., & Paita, L. M.
Article Title: Satisfaction with managed care
Journal Title: *Journal of Nursing Care Quality*
Volume (Issue): 15(1) **Year:** 2000 (October) **Pages:** 12–21

Summary: This article reports the findings of 1996, 1997, and 1998 patient satisfaction surveys administered to managed care enrollees in Utah. More than 14,000 managed care enrollees (both Medicaid and commercial) were selected randomly and contacted by telephone. The 38-question survey was based on Health Plan Employer Data and Information Set (HEDIS) and the National Committee for Quality Assurance (NCQA) measures. Demographic differences between the commercial and Medicaid population were identified. Medicaid enrollees were found to be higher users of health care services. Individuals reporting the greatest health plan satisfaction tended to be healthier. However, Medicaid enrollees reported greater overall health plan satisfaction than commercial enrollees.

Author(s): Pacala, J. T., Kane, R. L., Atherly, A. J., & Smith, M. A.
Article Title: Using structured implicit review to assess quality of care in the program of All-inclusive Care for the Elderly (PACE)
Journal Title: *Journal of the American Geriatrics Society*
Volume (Issue): 48(8) **Year:** 2000 (August) **Pages:** 903–910

Summary: To develop a quality assessment tool for care rendered to enrollees in the Program for All-inclusive Care of the Elderly (PACE) that can discriminate care quality ratings across PACE sites. Structured implicit review (SIR) of medical records by trained geriatricians and geriatric nurse-practitioners. Older adults enrolled in a PACE program for at least 6 months ($n = 313$). Overall care quality was judged to be above a community standard in 56% and below standard in 8% of cases. Process of care was rated as very good or good in 70% of the cases. Outcomes depended on how questions were phrased: only 19% of cases improved, whereas 28% were judged to have fared better than expected given their condition at baseline. Despite significant limitations of poor interrater reliability for process of care measures, excessive time involved for the reviews, and lack of a control group, the SIR method was able to consistently discriminate quality ratings among PACE sites. A modified version of the assessment instrument could prove useful in a quality improvement program for PACE care.

Author(s): Schifalacqua, M., Hook, M., O'Hearn, P., & Schmidt, M.
Article Title: Coordinating the care of the chronically ill in a world of managed care
Journal Title: *Nursing Administration Quarterly*
Volume (Issue): 24(3) **Year:** 2000 (Spring) **Pages:** 12–20

Summary: The systems required to provide coordinated health care to the chronically ill within a managed care contract are complex. As an integrated health care delivery system assuming shared financial risk of enrollees in a Medicare+ Choice contract, many care processes need to be created to meet the needs of the clients and administrators. Nursing case management and physician partnering are integral to the creation of the care model. The fiscal data demonstrated, for clients in the model, that there was an overall decrease in the inpatient length of stay, hospital days per thousand, and 30-day readmission rates.

Satisfaction with Care (N = 2)

Author(s): Oermann, M. H.
Article Title: Consumers' descriptions of quality health care
Journal Title: *Journal of Nursing Care Quality*
Volume (Issue): 14(1) **Year:** 1999 (October) **Pages:** 47–55

Summary: Consumer-oriented health care report cards have emerged as a strategy to disseminate information to consumers about the quality of health plans and relative costs, with the goal of enabling them to make informed choices. Although consumers have reported an interest in having access to this information, how they actually define quality of care is not yet clear. Despite extensive research on defining and measuring health care quality, less attention has been given to consumers' perspectives of quality care. In this study, 239 consumers were interviewed using four open-ended questions on their descriptions of quality health care and quality nursing care. Consumers described quality health care in terms of access to care ($n = 143$), followed by having competent and skilled providers ($n = 104$), and receiving the proper treatment ($n = 100$). Consumers defined quality nursing care as having nurses who were concerned about them and demonstrated caring behaviors ($n = 148$), were competent and skilled ($n = 115$), communicated effectively with them ($n = 99$), and taught them about their care ($n = 97$).

Author(s): Oermann, M. H., Lambert, J., & Templin, T.
Article Title: Parents' perceptions of quality health care
Journal Title: *MCN, American Journal of Maternal Child Nursing*
Volume (Issue): 25(5) **Year:** 2000 (September–October) **Pages:** 242–247

Summary: This was an exploratory study using a convenience sample of 229 consumers to examine differences in definitions of health care quality and the importance of indicators of quality. Important indicators of quality nursing care to parents with children were (1) being cared for by nurses who are up to date, well informed, and certified in their specialty; (2) being able to communicate with the nurse; (3) spending enough time with the nurse; and (4) teaching by the nurse. Although having access to midwives was of lowest importance to consumers overall, it was significantly more important to subjects with children ($p < .05$). Getting care and services when needed was also more important to parents than to consumers without children ($p = .05$). Parents gave more importance to their interactions with the nurse than did subjects without children ($t = 1.93$, df $= 229$, $p = .05$). Parents and consumers without children have similar views of what constitutes quality nursing care.

Quality Measurement and Nurse-Sensitive Outcomes: Sample Articles

9

Overview

This selected sample of articles was included so that nursing quality measurement efforts could be better understood in the context of the current health care delivery system. Important work on nurse-sensitive outcomes has continued to move forward during the last five years. The Nursing Outcomes Classification (NOC) completes the nursing process elements of the Nursing Minimum Data Set (NMDS) and provides standardized outcomes that can be used across the care continuum. The classification has a number of advantages, including being research-based, standardized, comprehensive, and flexible for clinical use. Another benefit of the NOC is that it enables inclusion of these data in data sets for health care effectiveness research (Maas, Mezey, & Harrington, 2000).

Also included is an important article summarizing the research priorities in areas of nurse staffing and nursing home quality (Kovner, Mezey, & Harrington, 2000). The authors maintain that nurse staffing and nursing home quality research should focus on resident outcomes instead of on nurses. In light of these discussions, it is clear that future quality measurement studies must incorporate patient outcomes as a key element of design and that a standardized classification strategy must be used that transcends all settings of care.

The seven articles in this chapter are organized as follows:

- Nursing outcomes classification
- Quality measurement and research priorities
- Nursing Interventions Classification (NIC) and Nursing Outcomes Classification (NOC)

Nursing Outcomes Classification (N = 4)

Author(s): Johnson, S. J., Brady-Schluttner K., Ellenbecker, S., Johnson, M., Lassegard, E., Maas, M., Stone, J. L., & Westra, B. L.

Article Title: Evaluating physical functional outcomes: One category of the NOC system
Journal Title: *MEDSURG Nursing*
Volume (Issue): 5(3) **Year:** 1996 (June) **Pages:** 157–162

Summary: All professional health care disciplines are now being held accountable to demonstrate the outcomes they produce. It is imperative that nurses demonstrate the difference they make in patient care to justify the cost of professional nursing. Standardized language is needed to aggregate data and report information on nursing interventions and associated outcomes. The Nursing Outcomes Classification (NOC) system is the first comprehensive classification of nursing-sensitive patient outcomes. In this review, the development of this classification system with specific results related to physical functional status and implications of NOC for nursing practice are discussed.

Author(s): Johnson, M., & Maas, M.
Article Title: The Nursing Outcomes Classification
Journal Title: *Journal of Nursing Care Quality*
Volume (Issue): 12(5) **Year:** 1998 (June) **Pages:** 9–20, 85–87

Summary: The NOC is a comprehensive taxonomy of patient outcomes influenced by nursing care. Each outcome is stated as a variable concept measured on a 5-point Likert scale and includes a definition, indicators, and references. The classification provides outcomes that can be used across the care continuum to assess patient status following nursing interventions. The classification has a number of advantages, including being research-based, standardized, comprehensive, and flexible for clinical use. It was developed by a large research team that included clinical experts, and has been subjected to testing.

Author(s): Maas, M. L., Johnson, M., & Moorhead, S.
Article Title: Classifying nursing-sensitive patient outcomes
Journal Title: *Image—the Journal of Nursing Scholarship*
Volume (Issue): 28(4) **Year:** 1996 (Winter) **Pages:** 295–301

Summary: This report describes research at the University of Iowa College of Nursing to develop a comprehensive classification of nursing-sensitive patient outcomes. The NOC completes the nursing process elements of the Nursing Minimum Data Set (NMDS). Resolution of conceptual and methodological problems that define the inductive approach taken to develop the NOC are described. Strategies used to develop NOC included review of the literature, clinical databases, and instruments; concept analysis; and surveys of nurse experts. Examples of outcomes, definitions, and indicators are presented. The NOC provides standardized patient outcomes for determining the effectiveness of nursing interventions and enables inclusion of these data in data sets for health care effectiveness research.

Author(s): Scherb, C. A., Rapp, C. G., Johnson, M., & Maas, M.
Article Title: The Nursing Outcomes Classification: Validation by rehabilitation nurses

Journal Title: *Rehabilitation Nursing*
Volume (Issue): 23(4)   **Year:** 1998 (July–August)   **Pages:** 174–178, 191

Summary: Measuring patient outcomes is important to rehabilitation nurses and the patients they serve. This article describes research conducted at the University of Iowa College of Nursing to develop the NOC and the validation of this research by surveys conducted through specialty nursing organizations, particularly the Association of Rehabilitation Nurses. Nurses responded to surveys designed to validate (a) the importance of outcome indicators to the achievement of an outcome, and (b) nursing's contribution to the achievement of the indicators. The results of the surveys indicate that rehabilitation nurses believe that nursing makes a substantial contribution to most outcomes and indicators.

Quality Measurement and Research Priorities (N = 2)

Author(s): Lancaster, D. R., & King, A.
Article Title: The spider diagram nursing quality report card: Bringing all the pieces together
Journal Title: *Journal of Nursing Administration*
Volume (Issue): 29(7/8)   **Year:** 1999 (July–August)   **Pages:** 43–48

Summary: The proliferation of information about nurse-sensitive quality outcome measures in the current data-driven health care environment can be overwhelming. Effective utilization of such data is an even greater challenge. In this article, the authors describe how the use of a spider diagram can serve to combine data from various sources into more meaningful information for decision making. This innovative quality report card format helps nurse executives to quickly gain an understanding of the interrelationships among existing structure, process, and outcome quality indicators, as well as to identify actual or potential quality-of-care issues.

Author(s): Kovner, C., Mezey, M., & Harrington, C.
Article Title: Research priorities for staffing, case mix, and quality of care in U.S. nursing homes
Journal Title: *Journal of Nursing Scholarship*
Volume (Issue): 32(1)   **Year:** 2000   **Pages:** 77–80

Summary: To inform the public about staffing and quality in nursing homes, the Hartford Institute for Geriatric Nursing convened a 1-day conference of 30 nurses, physicians, and other health professionals. This article summarizes research priorities in areas of nurse staffing and nursing home quality. In addition to specific research priorities, conference participants raised questions about research on nurse staffing and quality care. Several participants suggested that the research should focus on resident outcomes instead of on nurses. Participants addressed research priorities at resident, facility, and cross-facility levels. In all locations, case mix must be taken into account when studying any problem. Participants agreed that using OSCAR data requires understanding of its reliability and validity.

Nursing Interventions Classification (NIC) and Nursing Outcomes Classification (NOC) (N = 1)

Author(s): Hajewski, C., Maupin, J. M., Rapp, D. A., Sitterding, M., & Pappas, J.
Article Title: Implementation and evaluation of nursing interventions classification
Journal Title: *Journal of Nursing Care Quality*
Volume (Issue): 12(5)   **Year:** 1998 (June)   **Pages:** 30–40

Summary: Nursing Interventions Classification (NIC) and NOC are recognized examples of standardized nursing languages used to describe the contribution nursing makes to patient care. Columbus Regional Hospital nursing leadership recognized the need to use standardized nursing interventions and nursing-sensitive patient outcomes to describe the unique contribution nursing makes to patient education. In collaboration with the University of Iowa, NIC/NOC languages were implemented in the development of a patient education plan for a clinical pathway population.

References for This Book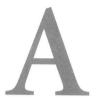

Adams, J., Kotarba, J. A., Wardell, D., Sherwood, G., Engebretson, J., & Salmon, L. (1996). An ethnographic assessment of an academic nursing center. *Journal of the American Academy of Nurse Practitioners, 8*(8), 365–371.

American Nurses Association. 1991. Task Force on Nursing Practice Standards and Guidelines: Working paper. *Journal of Nursing Quality Assurance, 5*(3), 1-17.

Alexander, G. L., & Stone, T. T. (2000). System review: A method for investigating medical errors in healthcare settings. *Nursing Case Management, 5*(5), 202–213.

Anderson, R. A., & McDaniel, R. R., Jr. (1999). RN participation in organizational decision making and improvements in resident outcomes. *Health Care Management Review, 24*(1), 7–16.

Anderson, R. A., Su, H., Hsieh, P., Allred, C. A., Owensby, S., & Joiner-Rogers, G. (1999). Case mix adjustment in nursing systems research: The case of resident outcomes in nursing homes. *Research in Nursing & Health, 22*(4), 271–283.

Aspling, D. L., & Lagoe, R. J. (1995). Development and implementation of a program to reduce hospital stays and manage resources on a community-wide basis. *Nursing Administration Quarterly, 20*(1), 1–11.

Banks, N., Palmer, R., Berwick, D., & Plsek, P. (1995). Variability in clinical systems: Applying modern quality control methods to health care. *The Joint Commission Journal on Quality Improvement, 21*(8), 407–417.

Barton, A. J., Danek, G., Johns, P., & Coons, M. (1998). Improving patient outcomes through CQI: Vascular access planning. *Journal of Nursing Care Quality, 13*(2), 77–85.

Bergenstal, R., Pearson, J., Cembrowski, G. S., Bina, D., Davidson, J., & List, S. (2000). Identifying variables associated with inaccurate self-monitoring of blood glucose: Proposed guidelines to improve accuracy. *Diabetes Educator, 26*(6), 981–989.

Blegen, M. A., & Vaughn, T. (1998). A multisite study of nurse staffing and patient occurrences. *Nursing Economics, 16*(4),196–203.

Blewitt, D. K., & Jones, K. R. (1996). Using elements of the nursing minimum data set for determining outcomes. *Journal of Nursing Administration, 26*(6), 48–56.

Bowers, B. J., Esmond, S., & Jacobson, N. (2000). The relationship between staffing and quality in long-term care facilities: exploring the views of nurse aides. *Journal of Nursing Care Quality, 4*(4), 55–64, 73–75.

Brickman, R., Axelrod, R., Roberson, D., & Flanagan, C. (1998). Clinical process improvement as a means of facilitating health care system integration. *Joint Commission Journal on Quality Improvement, 24*(3), 143–153.

Buonaccoro, K. M. (1999). Diabetic retinopathy screening: A clinical quality improvement project. *Journal for Healthcare Quality, 21*(6), 35–38.

Cole, F. L., Mackey, T., & Lindenberg, J. (1999). Search and research. Quality improvement: Psychometric evaluation of patient satisfaction with nurse practitioner care instrument. *Journal of the American Academy of Nurse Practitioners, 11*(11), 471–475.

Committee on Quality of Health Care in America (2001). *Crossing the quality chasm.* Washington, DC: Institute of Medicine, National Academy Press.

Committee on the National Quality Report on Health Care Delivery (2001). *Envisioning the national health care quality report.* Washington, DC: Institute of Medicine, National Academy Press.

Cox, R. A. (1998). Implementing nurse sensitive outcomes into care planning at a long-term care facility. *Journal of Nursing Care Quality, 12*(5), 41–51.

Derrick, A. M. (1998). Research corner. Benchmarking productivity in home health care. *Home Health Care Management & Practice, 10*(3), 71–77.

Donabedian, 1988 The quality of care: How can it be assessed? *Journal of the American Medical Association* September 23/30, 1988:260(12), 1743–1748.

Ellenbecker, C. H. (1995). Home health care industry growth and change: A study of one state's experience. *Home Health Care Services Quarterly, 15*(3), 61–81.

Ellenbecker, C. H., & Warren, K. (1998). Nursing practice and patient care in a changing home healthcare environment. *Home Healthcare Nurse, 16*(8), 531–539.

Elnitsky C., Nichols, B., & Palmer, K. (1997). Are hospital incidents being reported? *Journal of Nursing Administration, 27*(11), 40–46.

Flaherty, J. H., McBride, M., Marzouk, S. , Miller, D. K., Chien, N., Hanchett M,. Leander, S., Kaiser, F. E., & Morley, J. E. (1998). Decreasing hospitalization rates for older home care patients with symptoms of depression. *Journal of the American Geriatrics Society, 46*(1), 31–38.

Forbes, M. L., & Brown, H. N. (1995). Developing an instrument for measuring patient satisfaction. *AORN Journal, 61*(4), 737, 739, 741–743.

Franklin, P. D., & Legault, J. P. (1999). Using data to evaluate hospital inpatient mortality. *Journal of Nursing Care Quality, Special Issue* (no. 1), 55–66.

Frederick, P. R., Frankenfield, D. L., Biddle, M. G., & Sims, T. W. (1998). Changes in dialysis units' quality improvement practices from 1994 to 1996. *ANNA Journal, 25*(5), 469–478.

Fulmer, T. T., Feldman, P. H., Kim, T. S., Carty, B., Beers, M., Molina, M., & Putnam, M. (1999). An intervention study to enhance medication compliance in community-dwelling elderly individuals. *Journal of Gerontological Nursing, 25*(8), 6–14.

Gants, R. (1997). Detection and correction of underweight problems in nursing home residents. *Journal of Gerontological Nursing, 23*(12), 26–31.

Gardner, D.L. 1992. Measures of quality. In *Series on nursing administration: Volume III. Delivery of quality health care*, ed. M.Johnson and J.C. McCloskey, 42-58. St. Louis: Mosby Year Book.

Grobe, S. J., Becker, H., Calvin, A., Biering, P., Jordan, C., & Tabone, S. (1998). Clinical data for use in assessing quality: Lessons learned from the Texas Nurses' Association Report Card Project. *Seminars for Nurse Managers, 6*(3), 126–138.

Halfon, N., Newacheck, P. W., Hughes, D., & Brindis, C. (1998). Community health monitoring: Taking the pulse of America's children. *Maternal & Child Health Journal, 2*(2), 95–109.

Handler, A., Geller, S., & Kennelly, J. (1999). Effective MCH epidemiology in state health agencies: Lessons from an evaluation of the Maternal and Child Health Epidemiology Program (MCHEP). *Maternal & Child Health Journal, 3*(4), 217–224.

Harmon, R. L., Sheehy, L. M., & Davis, D. M. (1998). The utility of external performance measurement tools in program evaluation . . . presented, in part, at the annual meeting of the American Academy of Physical Medicine and Rehabilitation in Chicago in October 1996. *Rehabilitation Nursing, 23*(1), 8–11, 56.

Harrington, C., Zimmerman,D., Karon, S. L., Robinson, J., & Beutel, P. (2000). Nursing home staffing and its relationship to deficiencies. *Journals of Gerontology Series B-Psychological Sciences & Social Sciences, 55B*(5), S278–S287.

Harris-Wehling, J. 1990. Defining quality of care. In *Medicare: A strategy for quality assurance, Volume II. Sources and methods*, ed. K.N. Lohr, 116-139. Washington, DC: National Academy Press.

Hegyvary, S. T. 1991. Issues in outcomes research. *Journal of Nursing Quality Assurance.* 5(2), 1-6.

Hoare, K., Lacoste, J., Haro, K., & Conyers, C. (1999). Exploring indicators of telephone nursing quality. *Journal of Nursing Care Quality, 14*(1), 38–46.

Hoeffer, B., Rader, J., McKenzie, D., Lavelle, M., & Stewart, B. (1997). Reducing aggressive behavior during bathing cognitively impaired nursing home residents. *Journal of Gerontological Nursing, 23*(5), 16–23.

Johnson, M., Bulechek, G., McCloskey Dochterman, J., Maas, M., & Moorhead, S. (2001). *Nursing Diagnosis, Outcomes and Interventions: NANDA, NOC, and NIC Linkages*. St. Louis: Mosby.

Johnson, M., Maas, M. L., & Moorhead, S. (2000). *Nursing Outcomes Classification (NOC)* (2nd ed.). St. Louis: Mosby.

Johnson, M. & McCloskey, J.C. 1992. Quality in the nineties. In *Series on nursing administration: Volume III. Delivery of quality health care*, ed. M. Johnson and J.C. McCloskey, 59-68. St. Louis: Mosby Year Book.

Johnson-Pawlson, J., & Infeld, D. L. (1996). Nurse staffing and quality of care in nursing facilities. *Journal of Gerontological Nursing, 22*(8), 36–45.

Joint Commission on Accreditation of Healthcare Organizations (1998). *1998 standards for long term care*. Oakbrook Terrace, IL: the Author.

Joint Commission on Accreditation of Healthcare Organizations. (1990). *Accreditation manual for hospitals.* Chicago: the Author.

Joint Commission on Accreditation of Healthcare Organizations. (1992). *Accreditation manual for hospitals.* Oakbrook Terrace, IL: the Author.

Joint Commission on Accreditation of Healthcare Organizations. (1993). *Accreditation manual for hospitals.* Oakbrook Terrace, IL: the Author

Kangas, S., Kee, C. C., & McKee-Waddle, R. (1999). Organizational factors, nurses' job satisfaction, and patient satisfaction with nursing care. *Journal of Nursing Administration, 29*(1), 32–41.

Kansky, K. H., & Brannon, D. (1996). Discriminant analysis: A technique for adding value to patient satisfaction surveys. *Hospital & Health Services Administration, 41*(4), 503–513.

Katz, J. M., & Green, E. (1997). *Managing quality: A guide to system-wide performance management in health care* (2nd ed.). St. Louis: Mosby.

Kayser-Jones, J., & Schell, E. (1997). The mealtime experience of a cognitively impaired elder: Ineffective and effective strategies. *Journal of Gerontological Nursing, 23*(7), 33–39.

Knaus, V. L., Felten, S., Burton, S., Fobes, P., & Davis, K. (1997). The use of nurse practitioners in the acute care setting. *Journal of Nursing Administration, 27*(2), 20–27.

Koroknay, V. J., Werner, P., Cohen-Mansfield, J., & Braun, J. V. (1995). Maintaining ambulation in the frail nursing home resident: A nursing administered walking program. *Journal of Gerontological Nursing, 21*(11), 18–24.

Lang, N. M., Kraegel, J. M., Rantz, M. J., & Krejci, J. W. (1990). *Quality of health care for older people in America: A review of nursing studies.* Kansas City, MO: American Nurses Association.

Langner, S. R., & Hutelmyer, C. (1995). Patient satisfaction with outpatient human immunodeficiency virus care as delivered by nurse practitioners and physicians. *Holistic Nursing Practice, 10*(1), 54–60.

Larrabee, J. H., Ferri, J. A., & Hartig, M. T. (1997). Patient satisfaction with nurse practitioner care in primary care. *Journal of Nursing Care Quality, 11*(5), 9–14.

Lichtig, L. K., Knauf, R. A., & Milholland, D. K. (1999). Some impacts of nursing on acute care hospital outcomes. *Journal of Nursing Administration, 29*(2), 25–33.

Lowry, L. W., & Beikirch, P. (1998). Effect of comprehensive care on pregnancy outcomes . . . Ambulatory health care center for women and children called Genesis. *Applied Nursing Research, 11*(2), 55–61.

Luther, K. M., & Walsh, K. (1999). Moving out of the red zone: Addressing staff allocation to improve patient satisfaction. *Journal on Quality Improvement, 25*(7), 363–368.

Maas, M. L., Johnson, M., & Moorhead, S. (1996). Classifying nursing-sensitive patient outcomes. *Image—The Journal of Nursing Scholarship, 28*(4), 295–301.

Mackey, M. C., & Sobral. M. (1997). Staff evaluation of a high-risk pregnancy program. *Public Health Nursing, 14*(2), 101–110.

Marek, K. 1989. Outcome measurement in nursing. *Journal of Nursing Quality Assurance.* 4(1), 1-9.

McCloskey, J., & Bulechek, G. M. (2000). *Nursing Interventions Classification (NIC)* (3rd ed.). St. Louis: Mosby.

Meister, C., & Boyle, C. (1996). Perceptions of quality in long-term care: A satisfaction survey. *Journal of Nursing Care Quality, 10*(4), 40–47.

Miller, T.V. & Rantz, M.J. 1989. Management structures to facilitate practice changes subsequent to QA activities. *Journal of Nursing Quality Assurance, 3*(4), 21-27.

Minnick, A. F., & Pabst, M. K. (1998). Improving the ability to detect the impact of labor on patient outcomes. *Journal of Nursing Administration, 28*(12), 17–21.

Oermann, M. H., Dillon, S. L., & Templin, T. (2000). Indicators of quality of care in clinics: Patients' perspectives. *Journal for Healthcare Quality: Promoting Excellence in Healthcare, 22*(6), 9–12.

Oermann, M. H., & Templin, T. (2000). Important attributes of quality health care: Consumer perspectives. *Journal of Nursing Scholarship, 32*(2), 167–172.

Patyk, M., Gaynor, S., & Verdin, J. (2000). Patient education resource assessment: Project management. *Journal of Nursing Care Quality, 14*(2), 14–20.

Pearson, J. L., Lee, J. L., Chang, B. L., Elliott, M., Kahn, K. L., Rubenstein, & L. V. (2000). Structured implicit review: A new method for monitoring nursing care quality. *Medical Care, 38*(11), 1074–1091.

Rantz, M. J. (1995). *Nursing quality measurement: A review of nursing studies.* Washington, DC: American Nurses Association.

Rantz, M. J., Mehr, D. R., Conn, V. S., Hicks, L L., Porter, R., Madsen, R. W., Petroski, G. F., & Maas, M. (1996). Assessing quality of nursing home care: The foundation for improving resident outcomes. *Journal of Nursing Care Quality, 10*(4), 1–9.

Rantz, M. J, Petroski, G. F., Madsen, R. W., Scott, J., Mehr, D. R., Popejoy, L., Hicks, L. L., Porter, R., Zwygart-Stauffacher, M., & Grando, V. T. (1997). Setting thresholds for MDS quality indicators for nursing home quality improvement reports. *Journal of Quality Improvement, 23*(11), 602–611.

Rantz, M. J., Zwygart-Stauffacher, M., Popejoy, L., Grando, V. T., Mehr, D. R., Hicks, L. L., Conn, V. S., Wipke-Tevis, D., Porter, R., Bostick, J., & Maas, M. (1999). Nursing home care quality: A multidimensional theoretical model integrating the views of consumers and providers. *Journal of Nursing Care Quality, 14*(1), 16–37, 85–87.

Rantz, M. J., Petroski, G. F., Madsen, R.W., Mehr, D.R., Popejoy, L., Hicks, L. L., Porter, R., Zwygart-Stauffacher, M., & Grando, V. (2000a). Setting thresholds for quality indicators derived from MDS data for nursing home quality improvement reports: An update. *Journal on Quality Improvement, 26*(2), 101–110.

Rantz, M. J., Mehr, D. R., Petroski, G. F., Madsen, R. W., Popejoy, L L., Hicks, L L., Conn, V. S., Grando, V. T., Wipke-Tevis, D. D., Bostick, J., Porter, R., & Zwygart-Stauffacher, M., Maas, M. (2000b). Initial field testing of an instrument to measure: Observable indicators of nursing home care quality. *Journal of Nursing Care Quality, 14*(3), 1–12.

Redmond, G., Riggleman, J, Sorrell, J.M., & Zerull, L. (1999). Creative winds of change: Nurses collaborating for quality outcomes. *Nursing Administration Quarterly*, 23(2), 55–64.

Simmons, S. F., & Schnelle, J. F. (1999). Strategies to measure nursing home residents' satisfaction and preferences related to incontinence and mobility care: Implications for evaluating intervention effects. *Gerontologist, 39*(3), 345–355.

Singh, D. A., Amidon, R. L., Shi, L., & Samuels, M. E. (1996). Predictors of quality of care in nursing facilities. *Journal of Long Term Care Administration, 24*(3), 22–26.

Sochalski, J., Estabrooks, C. A., & Humphrey, C. K. (1999). Nurse staffing and patient outcomes: Evolution of an international study. *Canadian Journal of Nursing Research, 31*(3), 69–88.

Sorrell, J., & Redmond, G. (1997). Nursing Report Card Quality Indicator Project: Patients' stories of quality care. *Virginia Nurses Today, 5*(4), 10–11.

Steffen, T. M., & Nystrom, P. C. (1997). Validation of a measure of family members' perceptions of service quality in nursing homes. *Journal of Rehabilitation Outcomes Measurement, 1*(4), 1–9.

Strzalka, A., & Havens, D. S. (1996). Nursing care quality: Comparison of unit-hired, hospital float pool, and agency nurses. *Journal of Nursing Care Quality, 10*(4), 59–65.

Wakefield B., Buckwalter, K. C., & Collins, C. E. (1997). Assessing family satisfaction with care for persons with dementia. *Balance, 1*(1), 16–7, 40–42.

Wakefield, D. S., Hendryx , M. S., Uden-Holman, T., Couch, R., & Helms, C. M. (1996). Comparing providers' performance: problems in making the "report card" analogy fit. *Journal for Healthcare Quality: Promoting Excellence in Healthcare, 18*(6), 4–10.

Walker, P. H., Baker, J. J., & Chiverton, P. (1998). Costs of interdisciplinary practice in a school-based health center. *Outcomes Management for Nursing Practice, 2*(1), 37–44.

Waters, J. B., Wolff, R. S., Blansfield, J., LaMorte, W.W., Millham, F. H., & Hirsch, E. F. (1999). Development and implementation of clinical pathways for the management of four trauma diagnoses. *Journal for Healthcare Quality, 21*(3), 4–11.

Watson, C. J., Mobarak, A. M., & Stimson, K. (1999). A collaborative effort to establish a long-term care benchmark process. *Journal for Healthcare Quality, 21*(2), 19–23.

Glossary of Acronyms | B

ACE	Acute Care for Elders
ADL	activities of daily living
AHCPR	Agency for Health Care Policy and Research
AHOP	At Home Options Programs
AIDS	acquired immunodeficiency syndrome
ANA	American Nurses Association
APN	advanced practice nurses
APS	American Pain Society
BC	blood culture
BCNSEM	Blue Care Network of Southeast Michigan
CABG	coronary artery bypass graft
CBGM	capillary blood glucose monitoring
CHE	Catholic Health Ease
CHF	congestive heart failure
CMI	case mix indicator
CNO	community nursing organization
COPD	chronic obstructive pulmonary disease
CPS	cognitive performance scale
CQI	continuous quality improvement
CVL	central venous line
DKA	diabetic ketoacidosis
DNR	do not resuscitate
DRGs	diagnostic-related groups
ECF	extended care facility
ECG	electrocardiogram
ED	emergency department
EPPS	Enhanced Prospective Payment System
ESRD	end-stage renal disease
FADE	focus, analyze, develop, execute
FCDM	family caregiving dynamics model

FCPP	family-centered postpartum care
FFS	fee for service
GEM	geriatric evaluation and management
HCFA	Health Care Financing Administration
HCI	Holistic Caring Inventory
HCQIP	Health Care Quality Improvement Program
HEDIS	Health Plan Employer Data and Information Set
HHA	home health agencies
HIV	human immunodeficiency virus
HMO	health maintenance organization
IC	infection control
ICU	intensive care unit
IPC	Innovations in Patient Care
IV	intravenous
JCAHO	Joint Commission on Accreditation of Healthcare Organizations
LOS	length of stay
LTCF	long-term care facility
LWBS	leave without being seen (by a physician)
MAE	medication administration error
MCHEP	Maternal and Child Health Epidemiology Program
MDS	Minimum Data Set
MI	myocardial infarction
MISCHF	Management to Improve Survival in Congestive Heart Failure
MRSA	methicillin-resistant *Staphylococcus aureus*
MTX	methotrexate
NANDA	North American Nursing Diagnosis Association
NCNR	National Center for Nursing Research
NCQA	National Committee for Quality Assurance
NDNQI	National Database of Nursing Quality Indicators
NIC	nursing intervention classification
NICU	neonatal intensive care unit
NMDS	Nursing Minimum Data Set
NOC	Nursing Outcomes Classification
NP	nurse practitioner
NRMI	National Registry for Myocardial Infarction
OASIS	Outcome Assessment and Information Set
OBQI	Outcome-based quality improvement
OCP	outcome-focused care plans
OR	operating room
PACE	Program for All-inclusive Care of the Elderly
PC2000	Patient Care 2000
PEP	Practice Environment Program
PES	Program Evaluation System
PICU	pediatric intensive care unit
PIPC	Partners in Patient Care
POLST	Physician Orders for Life-Sustaining Treatment
POPM	patient opinion of pain management

PMP	pain management program
PRI	patient review instrument
PTCA	percutaneous transluminal coronary angioplasty
QA	quality assurance
QEC	quality of elder care
QHCQ	Quality Health Care Questionnaire
QIs	quality indicators
RAI	Resident Assessment Instrument
RAP	Resident Assessment Protocols
RDI	Referral Data Inventory
RN	registered nurse
RUGS III	Resource Utilization Groups III
SCU	special care unit
SDU	stepdown unit
SIMP-H	Schmele Instrument to Measure the Process of Nursing Practice in Home Health
SIR	structured implicit review
SMBG	self-monitoring of blood glucose
TDHS	Texas Department of Human Services
TPPC	traditional postpartum care
TPN	total parenteral nutrition
TQM	total quality management
UDS MR	Uniform Data System for Medical Rehabilitation
VAD	venous access device
VAMC	Veterans Affairs Medical Centers

Index of Citations | C

A

33 Adams, C. E., DeFrates, D. S., & Wilson, M. (1998). Data-driven quality improvement for HMO patients. *Journal of Nursing Administration, 28*(10), 20–25.

26 Adams, C. E., Kramer, S., & Wilson, M. (1995). Home health quality outcomes: Fee-for-service versus health maintenance organization enrollees. *Journal of Nursing Administration, 25*(11), 39–45.

33 Adams, C. E., Wilson, M., Haney, M., & Short, R. (1998). Using the outcome-based quality improvement model and OASIS to improve HMO patients' outcomes. *Home Healthcare Nurse, 16*(6), 395–401.

33 Adams, C. E., & Wilson, M. (1995). Enhanced quality through outcome-focused standardized care plans. *Journal of Nursing Administration, 25*(9), 27–34.

18 Adams, J., Kotarba, J. A., Wardell, D., Sherwood, G., Engebretson, J., & Salmon, L. (1996). An ethnographic assessment of an academic nursing center. *Journal of the American Academy of Nurse Practitioners, 8*(8), 365–371.

139 Agins, B., Young, M., Ellis, W., Burke, G., & Rotunno, F. (1995). A statewide program to evaluate the quality of care provided to persons with HIV infection. *The Joint Commission Journal on Quality Improvement, 21*(9), 439–456.

90 Aiken, L. H., Sloane, D. M., & Sochalski, J. (1998). Hospital organization and outcomes. *Quality in Health Care, 7*(4), 222–226.

54 Alcee, D. (2000). The experience of a community hospital in quantifying and reducing patient falls. *Journal of Nursing Care Quality, 14*(3), 43–53.

46 Alexander, G. L., & Stone, T. T. (2000). System review: A method for investigating medical errors in healthcare settings. *Nursing Case Management, 5*(5), 202–213.

20 Alexander, J., & Kroposki, M. (1999). Outcomes for community health nursing practice. *Journal of Nursing Administration, 29*(5), 49–56.

76 Anderson, M. A., & Helms, L. B. (1998). Extended care referral after hospital discharge. *Research in Nursing & Health, 21*(5), 385–394.

126 Anderson, R. A., Hsieh, P., & Su, H. (1998). Resource allocation and resident outcomes in nursing homes: Comparisons between the best and worst. *Research in Nursing & Health, 21*(4), 297–313.

126 Anderson, R. A., & McDaniel, R. R. Jr. (1999). RN participation in organizational decision making and improvements in resident outcomes. *Health Care Management Review, 24*(1), 7–16.

122 Anderson, R. A., Su, H., Hsieh, P., Allred, C. A., Owensby, S., & Joiner-Rogers, G. (1999). Case mix adjustment in nursing systems research: The case of resident outcomes in nursing homes. *Research in Nursing & Health, 22*(4), 271–283.

49   Anderson-Loftin, W., Wood, D., & Whitfield, L. (1995). A case study of nursing case management in a rural hospital. *Nursing Administration Quarterly, 19*(3), 33–40.

34   Arford P. H. Michel Y. McCue P. S., & Hiott, B. (1996). Quality and cost outcomes of transitional care. *Nursing Economics, 14*(5), 266–275.

49   Arford, P. H., & Allred, C. A. (1995). Value = quality + cost. *Journal of Nursing Administration, 25*(9), 64–69.

128 Arling, G., Karon, S. L. Sainfort, F., Zimmerman, D. R., & Ross, R. (1997). Risk adjustment of nursing home quality indicators. *Gerontologist, 37*(6), 757–766.

49   Aspling, D. L., & Lagoe, R. J. (1995). Development and implementation of a program to reduce hospital stays and manage resources on a community-wide basis. *Nursing Administration Quarterly, 20*(1), 1–11.

50   Ayestas, A. L. S., Diaz, E., & Kirtland, S. (1995). Clinical pathways: Improving patient education and influencing readmission rates. *Journal for Healthcare Quality, 17*(6), 17–25, 47.

B

134 Baer, W. M., & Hanson, L. C. (2000). Families' perception of the added value of hospice in the nursing home. *Journal of the American Geriatrics Society, 48*(8), 879–882.

90   Baggs, J. G., & Schmitt, M. H. (1997). Nurses' and resident physicians' perceptions of the process of collaboration in an MICU. *Research in Nursing & Health, 20*(1), 71–80.

50   Bailey, D. A., Litaker, D. G., & Mion, L. C. (1998). Developing better critical paths in healthcare: Combining 'best practice' and the quantitative approach. *Journal of Nursing Administration, 28*(7/8), 21–26.

101 Bailey, D. A., & Mion, L. C. (1997). Improving care givers' satisfaction with information received during hospitalization. *Journal of Nursing Administration, 27*(1), 21–27

54   Bankert, K., Daughtridge, S., Meehan, M., & Colburn, L. (1996). The application of collaborative benchmarking to the prevention and treatment of pressure ulcers. *Advances in Wound Care: The Journal for Prevention & Healing, 9*(2), 21–29.

17   Banks, N., Palmer, R., Berwick, D., & Plsek, P. (1995). Variability in clinical systems: Applying modern quality control methods to health care. *The Joint Commission Journal on Quality Improvement, 21*(8), 407–417.

94   Bantz, D., Wieseke, A., & Horowitz, J. (1995). 2,000 patients relate their hospital experiences. *Nursing Economics, 13*(6), 362–366.

46   Barton, A. J., Danek, G., Johns, P., & Coons, M. (1998). Improving patient outcomes through CQI: Vascular access planning. *Journal of Nursing Care Quality, 13*(2), 77–85.

122 Bell, P. A., & Smith, J. M. (1997). A behavior mapping method for assessing efficacy of change on special care units. *American Journal of Alzheimer's Disease, 12*(4), 184–189.

15   Bergenstal, R., Pearson, J., Cembrowski, G. S., Bina, D., Davidson, J., & List, S. (2000). Identifying variables associated with inaccurate self-monitoring of blood glucose: Proposed guidelines to improve accuracy. *Diabetes Educator, 26*(6), 981–989.

57   Bergh, I., & Sjostrom, B. (1999). A comparative study of nurses' and elderly patients' ratings of pain and pain tolerance. *Journal of Gerontological Nursing, 25*(5), 30–42.

114 Berlowitz, D. R., Ash, A. S., Brandeis, G. H., Brand, H. K., Halpern, J. L., & Moskowitz, M. A. (1996). Rating long-term care facilities on pressure ulcer development: Importance of case-mix adjustment. *Annals of Internal Medicine, 124*(6), 557–563.

114 Berlowitz, D. R., Bezerra, H. Q., Brandeis, G. H., Kader, B., & Anderson, J. J. (2000). Are we improving the quality of nursing home care: The case of pressure ulcers. *Journal of the American Geriatrics Society, 48*(1), 59–62.

61   Black, E. Weiss, K., Erban, S., & Shulkin, D. 1995. Innovations in patient care: Changing clinical practice and improving quality. *The Joint Commission Journal on Quality Improvement, 21*(8), 376–393.

101 Blackington, S. M., & McLauchlan, T. (1995). Continuous quality improvement in the neonatal intensive care unit: Evaluating parent satisfaction. *Journal of Nursing Care Quality, 9*(4), 78–85.

65   Blegen, M. A., & Vaughn, T. (1998). A multisite study of nurse staffing and patient occurrences. *Nursing Economics, 16*(4),196–203.

76   Blewitt, D. K., & Jones, K. R. (1996). Using elements of the nursing minimum data set for determining outcomes. *Journal of Nursing Administration, 26*(6), 48–56.

57   Bookbinder, M., Coyle, N., Kiss, M., Goldstein, M. L., Holritz, K., Thaler, H., Gianella, A., Derby, S., Brown, M., Racolin A., Ho, M. N., & Portenoy, R. K. (1996). Implementing national standards for cancer pain management: Program model and evaluation. *Journal of Pain & Symptom Management, 12*(6), 334–347.

34   Borchers, E. L. (1999). Improving nursing documentation for private-duty home health care. *Journal of Nursing Care Quality, 13*(5), 24–43, 91–92.

126 Bowers, B. J., Esmond, S., & Jacobson, N. (2000). The relationship between staffing and quality in long-term care facilities: Exploring the views of nurse aides. *Journal of Nursing Care Quality, 4*(4), 55–64, 73–75.

69   Brett, J. L., Bueno, M., Royal, N., & Kendall-Sengin, K. (1997). PRO-ACT II: Integrating utilization management, discharge planning, and nursing care management into the outcomes manager role. *Journal of Nursing Administration, 27*(2), 37–45.

46   Brickman, R., Axelrod, R., Roberson, D., & Flanagan, C. (1998). Clinical process improvement as a means of facilitating health care system integration. *Joint Commission Journal on Quality Improvement, 24*(3), 143–153.

77   Bromenshenkel, J., Newcomb, M., & Thompson, J. (2000). Continuous quality improvement efforts decrease postoperative ileus rates. *Journal for Healthcare Quality, 22*(2), 4–7.

73   Brooks, K., Whitten, S., & Quigley, D. (1998). Reducing the incidence of ventilator-related pneumonia. *Journal for Healthcare Quality, 20*(1), 14–19.

101 Bruce, T. A., Bowman, J. M., & Brown, S. T. (1998). Factors that influence patient satisfaction in the emergency department. *Journal of Nursing Care Quality, 13*(2), 31–37.

69   Bryan, Y. E., Hitchings, K. S., Fuss , M. A., Fox, M. A., Kinneman, M. T., & Young, M. J. (1998). Measuring and evaluating hospital restructuring efforts: Eighteen-month

follow-up and extension to critical care, part 1. *Journal of Nursing Administration, 28*(9), 21–27.

69 Bryan, Y. E., Hitchings, K. B., Fuss, M. A., Fox, M. A., Kinneman, M. T., & Young, M. J. (1998). Measuring and evaluating hospital restructuring efforts: Eighteen-month follow-up and extension to critical care, part 2. *Journal of Nursing Administration 28*(10), 13–19.

57 Buchanan, L., Voigtman, J., & Mills, H. (1997). Implementing the Agency for Health Care Policy and Research Pain Management Pediatric Guideline in a multicultural practice setting. *Journal of Nursing Care Quality, 11*(3), 23–35.

77 Bultema, J. K., Mailliard, L., Getzfrid, M. K., Lerner, R. D., & Colone, M. (1996). Geriatric patients with depression: Improving outcomes using a multidisciplinary clinical path model. *Journal of Nursing Administration, 26*(1), 31–38.

11 Buonaccoro, K. M. (1999). Diabetic retinopathy screening: A clinical quality improvement project. *Journal for Healthcare Quality, 21*(6), 35–38.

77 Burden, B., & Taft, E. (1999). A data-driven approach to improving clinical outcomes in cardiac care. *Journal for Healthcare Quality, 21*(2), 32–36.

16 Burma, M. R., Rachow, J. W., Kolluri, S., & Saag, K. G. (1996). Methotrexate patient education: A quality improvement study. *Arthritis Care & Research, 9*(3), 216–222.

86 Burris, G. W., & Jacobs, A. J. (1996). A continuous quality improvement process to increase organ and tissue donation. *Journal of Transplant Coordination, 6*(2), 88–92.

C

70 Cady, N., Mattes, M., & Burton, S. (1995). Reducing intensive care unit length of stay: A stepdown unit for first-day heart surgery patients. *Journal of Nursing Administration, 25*(12), 29–35.

58 Calvin, A., Becker, H., Biering, P., & Grobe, S. (1999). Measuring patient opinion of pain management. *Journal of Pain & Symptom Management, 8*(1), 17–26.

78 Card, S. J., Herrling, P. J., Matthews, J. L., Rossi, M. L., Spencer, E. S., & Lagoe, R. (1998). Impact of clinical pathways for total hip replacement: A community-based analysis. *Journal of Nursing Care Quality, 13*(2), 67–76.

78 Cardozo, L., & Aherns, S. (1999). Assessing the efficacy of a clinical pathway in the management of older patients hospitalized with congestive heart failure. *Journal for Healthcare Quality, 21*(3), 12–17.

54 Carey, R., & Teeters, J. (1995). CQI case study: Reducing medication errors. *The Joint Commission Journal on Quality Improvement, 21*(5), 233–237.

115 Carrol-Solomon, P. A., Christian, V., Denny, D. S., Nordan, V. N., Therriault, M. F., & Van Wisklen, R. (2000). Preserving residents' rights in long-term care settings: A values-based approach to restraint reduction. *Journal for Healthcare Quality, 22*(4), 10–19.

86 Carveth, J. A. (1995). Perceived patient deviance and avoidance by nurses. *Nursing Research, 44*(3), 173–178.

137 Castaneda-Mendez, K., Mangan, K., & Lavery, A. M. (1998). The role and application of the balanced scorecard in healthcare quality management. *Journal for Healthcare Quality, 20*(1), 10–13.

115 Castle, N. G. (2000). Deficiency citations for physical restraint use in nursing homes. *Journals of Gerontology Series B—Psychological Sciences & Social Sciences, 55B*(1), S33–S40.

116 Castle, N. G., & Fogel, B. (1998). Organizational structure and outcomes for nursing home residents with mental disorders. *Journal of Mental Health & Aging, 4*(1), 105–124.

58 Caswell, D. R., Williams, J. P, Vallejo, M., Zaroda, T., McNair, N., Keckeisen, M., Yale, C., & Cryer, H. G. (1996). Improving pain management in critical care. *Journal on Quality Improvement, 22*(10), 702–712.

58 Celia, B. (2000). Age and gender differences in pain management following coronary artery bypass surgery. *Journal of Gerontological Nursing, 26*(5), 7–13.

70 Chang, B. L., Rubenstein, L. V., Keeler, E. B., Miura, L. N., & Kahn, K. L. (1996). The validity of a nursing assessment and monitoring of signs and symptoms scale in ICU and non-ICU patients. *American Journal of Critical Care, 5*(4), 298–303.

106 Chewitt, M. D., Fallis, W. M., & Suski, M. C. (1997). The surgical hotline: Bridging the gap between hospital and home. *Journal of Nursing Administration, 27*(12), 42–49.

50 Chiverton, P., Tortoretti, D., LaForest, M., & Walker, P. H. (1999). Bridging the gap between psychiatric hospitalization and community care: Cost and quality outcomes. *Journal of the American Psychiatric Nurses Association, 5*(2), 46–53.

102 Clark, C. A., Pokorny, M. E., & Brown, S. T. (1996). Consumer satisfaction with nursing care in a rural community hospital emergency department. *Journal of Nursing Care Quality, 10*(2), 49–57.

90 Clark, L. R., Fraaza, V., Schroeder, S., & Maddens, M. E. (1995). Alternative nursing environments: Do they affect hospital outcomes? *Journal of Gerontological Nursing, 21*(11), 32–38.

20 Cleary, K. (1995). Using claims data to measure and improve the MMR immunization rate in an HMO. *The Joint Commission Journal on Quality Improvement, 21*(5), 211–217.

15 Cole, F. L., Mackey, T., & Lindenberg, J. (1999). Search and research. Quality improvement: Psychometric evaluation of patient satisfaction with nurse practitioner care instrument. *Journal of the American Academy of Nurse Practitioners, 11*(11), 471–475.

61 Counsell, S. R., Holder, C. M., Liebenauer, L. L., Palmer, R. M., Fortinsky, R. H., Kresevic, D. M., Quinn, L. M., Allen, K. R., Covinsky, K. E., & Landefeld, C. S. (2000). Effects of a multicomponent intervention on functional outcomes and process of care in hospitalized older patients: A randomized controlled trial of acute care for elders (ACE) in a community hospital. *Journal of the American Geriatrics Society, 48*(12), 1572–1581.

61 Covinsky, K. E., Palmer, R. M., Kresevic, D. M., Kahana, E., Counsell, S. R., Fortinsky, R. H., & Landefeld, C. S. (1998). Improving functional outcomes in older patients: Lessons from an acute care for elders unit. *Journal on Quality Improvement, 24*(2), 63–76.

116 Cox, R. A. (1998). Implementing nurse sensitive outcomes into care planning at a long-term care facility. *Journal of Nursing Care Quality, 12*(5), 41–51.

78 Crawley, W. D. (1996). Case management: Improving outcomes of care for ischemic stroke patients. *MEDSURG Nursing, 5*(4), 239–244.

51 Crawley, W. D., & Till, A. H. (1995). Case management: More population-based data. *Clinical Nurse Specialist, 9*(2), 116–120.

40 Cullen, D., Bates, D., Small, S. Cooper, J., Nemeskai, A., & Leape, L. (1995). The incident reporting system does not detect adverse drug events: A problem for quality improvement. *The Joint Commission Journal on Quality Improvement, 21*(10), 541–552.

35 Currie, G. A., Brofman, L., & Saharia, A. N. (1997). American Subacute Care Association. Outcomes-based home health care improves results for patients with CHF. *Home Care Provider, 2*(3), 143–147.

78 Cushing, K. A., & Stratta, R. J. (1997). Design, development, and implementation of a critical pathway in simultaneous pancreas-kidney transplant recipients. *Journal of Transplant Coordination, 7*(4), 164–172.

40 Czarnecki, M. T. (1996) . Benchmarking: A data-oriented look at improving health care performance. *Journal of Nursing Care Quality, 10*(3), 1–6.

D

58 Dalton, J. A., Blau, W., Lindley, C., Carlson, J., Youngblood, R., & Greer, S. M. (1999). Changing acute pain management to improve patient outcomes: An educational approach. *Journal of Pain & Symptom Management, 17*(4), 277–287.

35 Davis, J. H. (1996). Total parenteral nutrition (TPN) at home: Prototype high-tech home care nursing. *Gastroenterology Nursing, 19*(6), 207–209.

86 Dearborn, P., De Muth, J. S., Requarth, A. B., & Ward, S. E. (1997). Nurse and patient satisfaction with three types of venous access devices. *Oncology Nursing Forum, 24*(1 Suppl), 34–40.

40 Dearmin, B. J., Brenner, J., & Migliori, R. (1995). Reporting on QI efforts for internal and external customers. *The Joint Commission Journal on Quality Improvement, 21*(6), 277–288.

31 Derrick, A. M. (1998). Research corner. Benchmarking productivity in home health care. *Home Health Care Management & Practice, 10*(3), 71–77.

150 Donabedian, 1988 The quality of care: How can it be assessed? *Journal of the American Medical Association.* September 23/30, 1988:260(12), 1743–1748.

E

70 Effken, J. A., & Stetler, C. B. (1997). Impact of organizational redesign. *Journal of Nursing Administration, 27*(7/8), 23–32.

27 Ellenbecker, C.H. (1995). Profit and non-profit home health care agency outcomes: A study of one state's experience. *Home Health Care Services Quarterly, 15*(3), 47–60.

32 Ellenbecker, C. H. (1995). Home health care industry growth and change: A study of one state's experience. *Home Health Care Services Quarterly, 15*(3), 61–81.

29 Ellenbecker, C. H., & Warren, K. (1998). Nursing practice and patient care in a changing home healthcare environment. *Home Healthcare Nurse, 16*(8), 531–539.

141 Ellenbecker, C. H., Wagner, L., & Cloutterbuck, J. (1997). Using insurance claims data and medical record reviews to assess the quality of medical care. *Journal for Healthcare Quality, 19*(3), 21–31.

41 Elnitsky C., Nichols, B., & Palmer, K. (1997). Are hospital incidents being reported? *Journal of Nursing Administration, 27*(11), 40–46.

F

27 Flaherty, J. H., McBride, M., Marzouk, S., Miller, D. K., Chien, N., Hanchett M,. Leander, S., Kaiser, F. E., & Morley, J. E. (1998). Decreasing hospitalization rates for older home care patients with symptoms of depression. *Journal of the American Geriatrics Society, 46*(1), 31–38.

29   Foley, M. E., Fahs, M. C., Eisenhandler, J., & Hyer , K. (1995). Satisfaction with home healthcare services for clients with HIV: Preliminary findings. *Journal of the Association of Nurses in AIDS Care, 6*(5), 20–25.

15   Forbes, M. L., & Brown, H. N. (1995). Developing an instrument for measuring patient satisfaction. *AORN Journal, 61*(4), 737, 739, 741–743.

140   Forbes, S. A., Duncan, P, W., & Zimmerman, M. K. (1997). Review criteria for stroke rehabilitation outcomes. *Archives of Physical Medicine & Rehabilitation, 78*(10), 1112–1116.

41   Franklin, P. D., & Legault, J. P. (1999). Using data to evaluate hospital inpatient mortality. *Journal of Nursing Care Quality, Special Issue* (no. 1), 55–66.

11   Frederick, P. R., Frankenfield, D. L., Biddle, M,G., & Sims, T. W. (1998). Changes in dialysis units' quality improvement practices from 1994 to 1996. *ANNA Journal, 25*(5), 469–478.

65   Freer, Y., & Murphy-Black, T. (1995). Work rotas and performance levels: Evaluating the effects of twelve hour shifts against eight hour shifts on a neonatal intensive care unit. *Journal of Neonatal Nursing, 1*(4), 5–9.

133   Friedemann, M., Montgomery, R. J.. Maiberger, B., & Smith, A. A. (1997). Family involvement in the nursing home: Family-oriented practices and staff-family relations. *Research in Nursing & Health, 20*(6), 527–537.

65   Friedman C., & Chenoweth, C. (1998). A survey of infection control professional staffing patterns at University HealthSystem consortium institutions. *American Journal of Infection Control, 26*(3), 239–244.

27   Fulmer, T. T., Feldman, P. H., Kim, T. S., Carty, B., Beers, M., Molina, M., & Putnam, M. (1999). An intervention study to enhance medication compliance in community-dwelling elderly individuals. *Journal of Gerontological Nursing, 25*(8), 6–14.

71   Fuss, M. A., Bryan, Y. E,. Hitchings, K.S. , Fox, M.A., Kinneman, M. T., Skumanich, S., & Young, M. J. (1998). Measuring critical care redesign: Impact on satisfaction and quality. *Nursing Administration Quarterly, 23*(1), 1–14.

G

109   Galindo-Ciocon, D. J., Ciocon, J. O., & Galindo, D. J. (1995). Gait training and falls in the elderly. *Journal of Gerontological Nursing, 21*(6), 11–17.

117   Gants, R. (1997). Detection and correction of underweight problems in nursing home residents. *Journal of Gerontological Nursing, 23*(12), 26–31.

117   Gibson, C. J., Opalka, P. C, Moore, C. A., Brady, R. S., & Mion, L. C. (1995). Effectiveness of bran supplement on the bowel management of elderly rehabilitation patients. *Journal of Gerontological Nursing, 21*(10), 21–30.

13   Goode, C. J., Tanaka, D. J., Krugman, M., O'Connor, P. A., Bailey, P., Deutchman, M., & Stolpman, N. M. (2000). Outcomes from use of an evidence-based practice guideline. *Nursing Economics, 18*(4), 202–207.

51   Grant, P. H., Campbell, L. L., & Gautney, L. J. (1995). Implementing case management and developing clinical pathways. *Journal for Healthcare Quality, 17*(6), 10–16.

94   Gray, B. S. (1997). Focus group feedback from breast cancer patients. *Journal for Healthcare Quality, 19*(5), 32–36.

138   Green, P. L. (1998). Improving clinical effectiveness in an integrated care delivery system. *Journal for Healthcare Quality, 20*(6), 4–8.

79   Griffin H., Davis, L., Gant, E., Savona, M., Shaw, L., Strickland J., Wood, C., & Wagner,

G. (1999). A community hospital's effort to expedite treatment for patients with chest pain. *Heart & Lung: Journal of Acute & Critical Care, 28*(6), 402–408.

91   Grindel, C. G., Peterson, K. , Kinneman, M., & Turner, T. L. (1996). The Practice Environment Project: A process for outcome evaluation. *Journal of Nursing Administration, 26*(5), 43–51.

41   Grobe, S. J., Becker, H., Calvin, A., Biering, P., Jordan, C., & Tabone, S. (1998). Clinical data for use in assessing quality: Lessons learned from the Texas Nurses' Association Report Card Project. *Seminars for Nurse Managers, 6*(3), 126–138.

13   Gruber, J. L. (1999). Strategies for implementing quantifiable group practice guidelines. *Journal for Healthcare Quality, 21*(4), 11–20.

110   Gunn, S., Hanisch, P., & Wood, D. (1995). CQI action team: Responding to the detoxification patient. *The Joint Commission Journal on Quality Improvement, 21*(10), 531–540.

H

147   Hajewski, C., Maupin, J. M., Rapp, D. A., Sitterding, M., & Pappas, J. (1998). Implementation and evaluation of nursing interventions classification. *Journal of Nursing Care Quality, 12*(5), 30–40.

22   Halfon, N., Newacheck, P. W., Hughes, D., & Brindis, C. (1998). Community health monitoring: Taking the pulse of America's children. *Maternal & Child Health Journal, 2*(2), 95–109.

79   Hall, G. R., Karstens, M., Rakel, B., Swanson, E., & Davidson, A. (1995). Managing constipation using a research-based protocol. *MEDSURG Nursing, 4*(1), 11–20.

80   Hamilton, L., & Lyon, P. S. (1995). A nursing-driven program to preserve and restore functional ability in hospitalized elderly patients. *Journal of Nursing Administration, 25*(4), 30–37.

23   Handler, A., Geller, S., & Kennelly, J. (1999). Effective MCH epidemiology in state health agencies: Lessons from an evaluation of the Maternal and Child Health Epidemiology Program (MCHEP). *Maternal & Child Health Journal, 3*(4), 217–224.

66   Hansen, B. S., & Benitez, D. I. (2000). Quantified caring. *Nursing Administration Quarterly, 24*(4), 72–79.

34   Hanstine, S., & Fanning, V. (2000). Teaching patients to manage diabetes safely in the home. *Home Health Care Management & Practice, 12*(4), 40–48.

47   Harmon, R. L., Sheehy, L. M., & Davis, D. M. (1998). The utility of external performance measurement tools in program evaluation . . . presented, in part, at the annual meeting of the American Academy of Physical Medicine and Rehabilitation in Chicago in October 1996. *Rehabilitation Nursing, 23*(1), 8–11, 56.

127   Harrington, C., Zimmerman, D., Karon, S. L., Robinson, J., & Beutel, P. (2000). Nursing home staffing and its relationship to deficiencies. *Journals of Gerontology Series B—Psychological Sciences & Social Sciences, 55B*(5), S278–S287.

87   Harris, J. L., & Maguire, D. (1999). Developing a protocol to prevent and treat pediatric central venous catheter occlusions. *Journal of Intravenous Nursing, 22*(4), 194–198.

94   Harrison, E. (1995). Nurse caring and the new health care paradigm. *Journal of Nursing Care Quality, 9*(4), 14–23.

117   Hasel, K. L., & Erickson, R. S. (1995). Effect of cerumen on infrared ear temperature measurement. *Journal of Gerontological Nursing, 21*(12), 6–14.

102 Haynie, L., & Garrett, B. (1999). Developing a customer-service and cost-effectiveness team. *Journal for Healthcare Quality, 21*(6), 28–34.

12 Hearn, K., Dailey, M., Harris, M. T., & Bodian, C. (2000). Reduce costs and improve patient satisfaction with home pre-operative bowel preparations. *Nursing Case Management, 5*(1), 13–25.

80 Heckman, M., Ajdari, S. Y., Esquivel, M., Chernof, B., Tamm, N., Landowski, L., & Guterman, J. J. (1998). Quality improvement principles in practice: The reduction of umbilical cord blood errors in the labor and delivery suite. *Journal of Nursing Care Quality, 12*(3), 47–54.

62 Heinemann, D., Lengacher, C. A., VanCott, M. L., Mabe, P., & Swymer, S. (1996). Partners in patient care: Measuring the effects on patient satisfaction and other quality indicators. *Nursing Economics, 14*(5), 276–285.

131 Heliker, D. M. (1997). A narrative approach to quality care in long-term care facilities. *Journal of Holistic Nursing, 15*(1), 68–81.

106 Henzler, C., & Harper, J. (1995). Implementing a computer-assisted appropriateness review using DRG 182/183. *The Joint Commission Journal on Quality Improvement, 21*(5), 239–247.

73 Herchline, T., & Gros, S. (1997). Implementation of consensus guidelines for the follow-up of positive blood cultures. *Infection Control & Hospital Epidemiology, 18*(1), 38–41.

87 Hill, M. G., Fieselmann, J. F., Nobiling, H. E., O'Neill, P. S., Barry-Walker, J., Dwyer, J., & Kobler, L. (1995). Preventing cardiopulmonary arrest via enhanced vital signs monitoring. *MEDSURG Nursing, 4*(4), 289–95.

17 Hoare, K., Lacoste, J., Haro, K., & Conyers, C. (1999). Exploring indicators of telephone nursing quality. *Journal of Nursing Care Quality, 14*(1), 38–46.

123 Hoeffer, B., Rader, J., McKenzie, D., Lavelle, M., & Stewart, B. (1997). Reducing aggressive behavior during bathing cognitively impaired nursing home residents. *Journal of Gerontological Nursing, 23*(5),16–23.

110 Holle, M. L., Rick, C., Sliefert, M. K., & Stephens, K. (1995). Integrating patient care delivery. *Journal of Nursing Administration, 25*(7/8), 32–37.

117 Holtzman J., Degelau, J., Meyers, R., Christianson, C., & Lurie, N. (1997). Development and testing of a process measure of nursing home quality of care. *Journal of the American Geriatrics Society, 45*(10), 1203–1207.

80 Homes, L. M., & Hollabaugh, S. K. (1997). Using the continuous quality improvement process to improve the care of patients after angioplasty. *Critical Care Nurse, 17*(6), 56–60, 62–65.

20 Honnas, R., & Zlotnick, C. (1995). Quality improvement in action: Development of a tool. *Journal of Nursing Care Quality, 9*(4), 72–77.

54 Hopkins, B., Hanlon, M., Yauk, S., Sykes, S., & Rose, T. (2000). Reducing nosocomial pressure ulcers. *Journal of Nursing Care Quality, 14*(3), 28–36.

12 Horowitz, C. R., Goldberg, H. I., Martin, D. P., Wagner, E. H., Fihn, S. D., Christensen, D. B., & Cheadle, A. D. (1996). Conducting a randomized controlled trial of CQI and academic detailing to implement clinical guidelines. *Journal on Quality Improvement, 22*(11), 734–750.

94 Hostutler, J. J., Taft, S. H., & Snyder, C. (1999). Patient needs in the emergency department. *Journal of Nursing Administration, 29*(1), 43–50.

55 Huda, A., & Wise, L. C. (1998). Evolution of compliance within a fall prevention program. *Journal of Nursing Care Quality, 12*(3), 55–63.

95   Hunter, M. A., & Larrabee, J. H. (1998). Women's perceptions of quality and benefits of postpartum care. *Journal of Nursing Care Quality, 13*(2), 21–30.

I

141   Ipsen, S. K., Fosbinder, D., Williams, M., Warnick, M., Lertwachara, K., & Paita, L. M. (2000). Satisfaction with managed care. *Journal of Nursing Care Quality, 15*(1), 12–21.

51   Ireson C. L. (1997). Critical pathways: Effectiveness in achieving patient outcomes. *Journal of Nursing Administration, 27*(6), 16–23.

J

88   Jackson, G., & Andrew, J. (1996). Using a multidisciplinary CQI approach to reduce ER-to-floor admission time. *Journal for Healthcare Quality, 18*(3), 18–21.

102   Jacox, A. K., Bausell, B. R., & Mahrenholz, D. M. 1997. Patient satisfaction with nursing care in hospitals. *Outcomes Management for Nursing Practice, 1*(1), 20–28.

138   Jennings, B. M., & Staggers, N. (1999). A provocative look at performance measurement. *Nursing Administration Quarterly, 24*(1), 17–30.

32   Jette, A. M., Smith, K. W., & McDermott, S. M. (1996). Quality of Medicare-reimbursed home health care. *Gerontologist, 36*(4), 492–501.

146   Johnson, M., & Maas, M. (1998). The Nursing Outcomes Classification. *Journal of Nursing Care Quality, 12*(5), 9–20, 85–87.

145   Johnson, S. J., Brady-Schluttner, K., Ellenbecker, S., Johnson, M, Lassegard, E., Maas, M., Stone, J. L., & Westra, B. L. (1996). Evaluating physical functional outcomes: One category of the NOC system. *MEDSURG Nursing, 5*(3), 157–162.

127   Johnson-Pawlson, J., & Infeld, D. L. (1996). Nurse staffing and quality of care in nursing facilities. *Journal of Gerontological Nursing, 22*(8), 36–45.

62   Jones, R. A. P., Dougherty, M., & Martin, S. (1997). Program evaluation of a unit reengineered for patient-focused care. *Holistic Nursing Practice, 11*(3), 31–46.

95   Jones, K. R., Burney, R. E., & Christy, B. (2000). Patient expectations for surgery: Are they being met? *Journal on Quality Improvement, 26*(6), 349–360.

140   Jones, M. E., & Bond, M. L. (1999). Predictors of birth outcome among Hispanic immigrant women. *Journal of Nursing Care Quality, 14*(1), 56–62.

K

28   Kane, R. A., Frytak, J., & Eustis, N. N. (1997). Agency approaches to common quality problems in home care: A scenario study. *Home Health Care Services Quarterly, 16*(1/2), 21–40.

95   Kangas, S., Kee, C. C., & McKee-Waddle, R. (1999). Organizational factors, nurses' job satisfaction, and patient satisfaction with nursing care. *Journal of Nursing Administration, 29*(1), 32–41.

30   Kansky, K. H., & Brannon, D. (1996). Discriminant analysis: A technique for adding value to patient satisfaction surveys. *Hospital & Health Services Administration, 41*(4), 503–513.

118   Kayser-Jones, J. (1997). Inadequate staffing at mealtime: Implications for nursing and health policy. *Journal of Gerontological Nursing, 23*(8), 14–21.

118   Kayser-Jones, J., & Schell, E. (1997). The mealtime experience of a cognitively impaired elder: Ineffective and effective strategies. *Journal of Gerontological Nursing, 23*(7), 33–39.

103 Kellar, N., Martinez, J., Finnis, N., Bolger, A., & von Gunten, C. F. (1996). Characterization of an acute impatient hospice palliative care unit in a U.S. teaching hospital. *Journal of Nursing Administration, 26*(3), 16–20.

28 Kendra, M. A., & Weiker, A. (1996). Chart audit using the American Nurses Association standards of practice. *Home Healthcare Nurse, 14*(7), 551–556.

30 Kendra, M. A., Weiker, A., Simon, S., Grant, A., & Shullick, D. (1996). Safety concerns affecting delivery of home health care. *Public Health Nursing, 13*(2), 83–89.

96 Kirchhoff, K. T., & Beckstrand, R. L. (2000). Critical care nurses' perceptions of obstacles and helpful behaviors in providing end-of-life care to dying patients. *American Journal of Critical Care, 9*(2), 96–105.

66 Knaus, V. L., Felten, S., Burton, S., Fobes, P., & Davis, K. (1997). The use of nurse practitioners in the acute care setting. *Journal of Nursing Administration, 27*(2), 20–27.

103 Koman, A. R., Kunik, M. E., Molinari, V., Ponce, H. , Rezabek, P., & Orengo, C. A. (1999). Discharge plans from a geropsychiatric unit: Patient and family satisfaction. *Clinical Gerontologist, 20*(4), 29–38.

119 Koroknay, V. J., Werner, P., Cohen-Mansfield, J., & Braun, J. V. (1995). Maintaining ambulation in the frail nursing home resident: A nursing administered walking program. *Journal of Gerontological Nursing, 21*(11), 18–24.

119 Kovach, C. R., & Henschel, H. (1996). Planning activities for patients with dementia: A descriptive study of therapeutic activities on special care units. *Journal of Gerontological Nursing, 22*(9), 33–38.

147 Kovner, C., Mezey, M., & Harrington, C. (2000). Research priorities for staffing, case mix, and quality of care in U.S. nursing homes. *Journal of Nursing Scholarship, 32*(1), 77–80.

138 Kroll, D. A., Brummitt, C. F., & Berry, B. B. (2000). A users group approach to quality improvement across an integrated healthcare delivery system. *Journal for Healthcare Quality, 22*(1), 39–43.

119 Kuehn, A. F., & Sendelweck, S. (1995). Acute health status and its relationship to falls in the nursing home. *Journal of Gerontological Nursing, 21*(7), 41–49.

L

42 Lagoe, R. J., Noetscher, C. M., & Murphy, M. E. (2000). Hospital readmissions at the community level: Implications for case management. *Journal of Nursing Care Quality, 14*(4), 1–15.

42 Lagoe, R. J., Noetscher, C. M., & Murphy, M. E. (2000). Combined benchmarking of hospital outcomes and utilization. *Nursing Economics, 18*(2), 63–70.

42 Lagoe, R. J., Noetscher, C. M., Hohner, V. K., & Schmidt, G. M. (1999). Analyzing hospital readmissions using statewide discharge databases. *Journal of Nursing Care Quality, 13*(6), 57–67.

23 Lamb, G. S. (1995). Early lessons from a capitated community-based nursing model. *Nursing Administration Quarterly, 19*(3), 18–26.

147 Lancaster, D. R., & King, A. (1999). The spider diagram nursing quality report card: Bringing all the pieces together. *Journal of Nursing Administration, 29*(7/8), 43–48.

14 Langner, S. R., & Hutelmyer, C. (1995). Patient satisfaction with outpatient human immunodeficiency virus care as delivered by nurse practitioners and physicians. *Holistic Nursing Practice, 10*(1), 54–60.

14 Larrabee, J. H., Ferri, J. A., & Hartig, M. T. (1997). Patient satisfaction with nurse practitioner care in primary care. *Journal of Nursing Care Quality, 11*(5), 9–14.

28   Lee, T. T., & Mills, M. E. (2000). Analysis of patient profile in predicting home care resource utilization and outcomes. *Journal of Nursing Administration, 30*(2), 67–75.

21   Leff, E., Schriefer, J., Hagan, J., & DeMarco, P. (1995). Improving breastfeeding support: A community health improvement project. *The Joint Commission Journal on Quality Improvement, 21*(10), 521–529.

91   Leppa, C. J. (1996). Nurse relationships and work group disruption. *Journal of Nursing Administration, 26*(10), 23–27.

91   Leveck, M. L., & Jones, C. B. (1996). The nursing practice environment, staff retention, and quality of care. *Research in Nursing & Health, 19*(4), 331–343.

66   Lichtig, L. K., Knauf, R. A., & Milholland, D. K. (1999). Some impacts of nursing on acute care hospital outcomes. *Journal of Nursing Administration, 29*(2), 25–33.

31   Litherland, K. (1995). Lessons learned while implementing service quality improvement. *Journal for Healthcare Quality, 17*(5), 14–17.

52   Little, A. B., & Whipple, T. W. (1996). Clinical pathway implementation in the acute care hospital setting. *Journal of Nursing Care Quality, 11*(2), 54–61.

12   Lowry, L. W., & Beikirch, P. (1998). Effect of comprehensive care on pregnancy outcomes . . . ambulatory health care center for women and children called Genesis. *Applied Nursing Research, 11*(2), 55–61.

66   Luther, K. M., & Walsh, K. (1999). Moving out of the red zone: Addressing staff allocation to improve patient satisfaction. *Journal on Quality Improvement, 25*(7), 363–368.

52   Lynn, M. R., & Kelley, B. (1997). Effects of case management on the nursing context—perceived quality of care, work satisfaction, and control over practice. *Image—The Journal of Nursing Scholarship, 29*(3), 237–241.

96   Lynn, M. R., & McMillen, B. J. (1999). Do nurses know what patients think is important in nursing care? *Journal of Nursing Care Quality, 13*(5), 65–74.

96   Lynn, M. R., & Moore, K. (1997). Relationship between traditional quality indicators and perceptions of care. *Seminars for Nurse Managers, 5*(4), 187–193.

140   Lynne, J., Schall, M. W., Milne, C., Nolan, K. M., & Kabcenell, A. (2000). Quality improvements in end of life care: Insights from two collaboratives. *Journal on Quality Improvement, 26*(5), 254–267.

M

146   Maas, M. L., Johnson, M., & Moorhead, S. (1996). Classifying nursing–sensitive patient outcomes. *Image - the Journal of Nursing Scholarship, 28*(4), 295–301.

73   Mabon, B. L., Ciardi, B., Nouri, K., & Ruben, F. L. (1997). Concise communications. Skin testing for tuberculosis in university teaching hospitals—is there a problem? *Infection Control & Hospital Epidemiology, 18*(4), 247–249.

13   Mackey, M. C., & Sobral, M. (1997). Staff evaluation of a high-risk pregnancy program. *Public Health Nursing, 14*(2), 101–110.

92   Malloch K. (2000). Healing models for organizations: Description, measurement, and outcomes. *Journal of Healthcare Management, 45*(5), 332–346.

35   Malnory, M. (1997). Mother-infant home care drives quality in a managed care environment. *Journal of Nursing Care Quality, 11*(4), 9–26.

129   Marek, K. D., Rantz, M. J., Fagin, C. M., & Krejci, J. W. (1996). OBRA '87: Has it resulted in better quality of care? *Journal of Gerontological Nursing, 22*(10), 28–36.

71   Marino, B. L., & Ganser, C. C. (1997). Sensitivity of patient report of care to organizational change. *Journal of Nursing Administration, 27*(4), 32–36.

43   Mark, B. A., & Burleson, D. L. (1995). Measurement of patient outcomes: Data availability and consistency across hospitals. *Journal of Nursing Administration, 25*(4), 52–59.

81   Maxey, C. (1997). A case map reduces time to administration of thrombolytic therapy in patients experiencing an acute myocardial infarction. *Nursing Case Management, 2*(5), 229–237.

88   McArthur, C. L. III, & Rooke, C. T. (1995). Are spinal precautions necessary in all seizure patients? . . . presented at SAEM, Toronto, May 1992. *American Journal of Emergency Medicine, 13*(5), 512–513.

43   McKay, M. D., Rowe, M. M., & Bernt, F. M. (1997). Disease chronicity and quality of care in hospital readmissions. *Journal for Healthcare Quality, 19*(2), 33–36.

81   Meier, P. P., Engstrom, J. L,. Fleming, B. A., Streeter , P. L., & Lawrence, P. B. (1996). Estimating milk intake of hospitalized preterm infants who breastfeed. *Journal of Human Lactation, 12*(1), 21–26.

132   Meister, C., & Boyle, C. (1996). Perceptions of quality in long-term care: A satisfaction survey. *Journal of Nursing Care Quality, 10*(4), 40–47.

129   Mentes, J., Culp, K., Maas, M., & Rantz, M. (1999). Acute confusion indicators: Risk factors and prevalence using MDS data. *Research in Nursing & Health, 22*(2), 95–105.

88   Miller, K. D., & Deitrick, C. L. (1997). Experience with PICC at a University Medical Center [corrected] [published erratum appears in *J Intravenous Nurs* 1997 Jul–Aug; 20(4), 206]. *Journal of Intravenous Nursing, 20*(3), 141–147.

62   Miller, D., Smith, D. J., Brophy, M., Mollman, M., Owen, J., Smith, G., & More, C. (1996). Total quality improvement: An example of an effective team. *Journal for Healthcare Quality, 18*(1), 20–23.

67   Minnick, A. F., & Pabst, M. K. (1998). Improving the ability to detect the impact of labor on patient outcomes. *Journal of Nursing Administration, 28*(12), 17–21.

55   Minnick, A. F., Mion, L. C., Leipzig, R., Lamb, K., & Palmer, R. M. (1998). Prevalence and patterns of physical restraint use in the acute care setting. *Journal of Nursing Administration, 28*(11), 19–22.

72   Mitchell, P. H., Shannon, S. E., Cain, K. C., & Hegyvary, S. (1996). Critical care outcomes: Linking structures, processes, and organizational and clinical outcomes. *American Journal of Critical Care, 5*(5), 353–365.

43   Moore, K., Lynn, M. R., McMillen, B. J., & Evans S. (1999). Implementation of the ANA report card. *Journal of Nursing Administration, 29*(6), 48–54.

14   Morishita, L., Boult, C., Boult, L., Smith, S., & Pacala, J. T. (1998). Satisfaction with outpatient geriatric evaluation and management (GEM). *Gerontologist, 38*(3), 303–308.

21   Morriey-Ro, M., & Greiner, P. A. (2000). Hitting the mark in community health outreach: What counts? *Journal for Healthcare Quality, 22*(1), 17–23.

110   Mosley, A., Galindo-Ciocon, D., Peak, N., & West, M. J. (1998). Initiation and evaluation of a research-based fall prevention program. *Journal of Nursing Care Quality, 13*(2), 38–44.

123   Mukamel, D. B., & Brower, C. A. (1998). The influence of risk adjustment methods on conclusions about quality of care in nursing homes based on outcome measures. *Gerontologist, 38*(6), 695–703.

74   Murphy, M., Noetscher, C., & Lagoe, R. (1999). A multihospital effort to reduce inpatient lengths of stay for pneumonia. *Journal of Nursing Care Quality, 13*(5), 11–23.

119   Mylotte, J. M. (1996). Measuring antibiotic use in a long-term care facility. *American Journal of Infection Control, 24*(3), 174–179.

N

106   Nahm, R., & Poston, I. (2000). Measurement of the effects of an integrated, point-of-care computer system on quality of nursing documentation and patient satisfaction. *Computers in Nursing, 18*(5), 220–229.

63   Nardone, P. L., Markie, J. W., & Tolle, S. (1995). Evaluating a nursing care delivery model using a quality improvement design. *Journal of Nursing Care Quality, 10*(1), 70–84.

63   Nash, M. G., Grant, J. S., & Bartolucci, A. A. (2000). Clinical and operational outcomes of a work redesign model. *National Academies of Practice Forum: Issues in Interdisciplinary Care (NAPF), 2*(3), 203–210.

74   Nicotra, D., & Ulrich, C. (1996). Process improvement plan for the reduction of nosocomial pneumonia in patients on ventilators. *Journal of Nursing Care Quality, 10*(4), 18–23.

96   Niedz, B. A. (1998). Correlates of hospitalized patients' perceptions of service quality. *Research in Nursing & Health, 21*(4), 339–349.

O

16   Oakley, D., & Bogue, E. (1995). Quality of condom use as reported by female clients of a family planning clinic. *American Journal of Public Health, 85*(11),1526–1530.

97   O'Connor, S. J., Trinh, H. Q., & Shewchuk, R. M. (2000). Perceptual gaps in understanding patient expectations for health care service quality. *Health Care Management Review, 25*(2), 7–23.

142   Oermann, M. H. (1999). Consumers' descriptions of quality health care. *Journal of Nursing Care Quality, 14*(1), 47–55.

10   Oermann, M. H., Dillon, S. L., & Templin, T. (2000). Indicators of quality of care in clinics: Patients' perspectives. *Journal for Healthcare Quality: Promoting Excellence in Healthcare, 22*(6), 9–12.

143   Oermann, M. H., Lambert, J., & Templin, T. (2000). Parents' perceptions of quality health care. *MCN, American Journal of Maternal Child Nursing, 25*(5), 242–247.

10   Oermann, M. H., & Templin, T. (2000). Important attributes of quality health care: Consumer perspectives. *Journal of Nursing Scholarship, 32*(2),167–172.

139   Oermann, M. H., & Wilson, F. L. (2000). Quality of care information for consumers on the Internet. *Journal of Nursing Care Quality, 14*(4), 45–54.

81   Oetker, D., & Cole, C. (1996). Improving the outcome of emergency department patients with a chief complaint of chest pain. *Journal of Nursing Care Quality, 10*(2), 58–74.

44   Olt, F., Wilson, D., Ron, A., & Soffel, D. (1997). Quality improvement through review of inpatient deaths. *Journal for Healthcare Quality, 19*(1), 12–18.

97   Owens, R., & Cronin, S. N. (1998). Nurses' attitudes towards cost-effectiveness and quality of care. *Cost & Quality Quarterly Journal, 4*(3), 18–22.

P

142 Pacala, J. T., Kane, R. L., Atherly, A. J., & Smith, M. A. (2000). Using structured implicit review to assess quality of care in the program of All-inclusive Care for the Elderly (PACE). *Journal of the American Geriatrics Society, 48*(8), 903–910.

59 Paice, J., Mahon, S. M., & Faut-Callahan, M. (1995). Pain control in hospitalized post-surgical patients. *MEDSURG Nursing, 4*(5), 367–372.

82 Painter, L. M., Dudjak, L. A., Breiner, K., & Langford, A. (1995). Abdominal aortic aneurysm pathway: Outcome analysis. *Journal of Vascular Nursing, 13*(4), 101–105.

123 Pandolph, A., Mazzoni-Maddigan, J. , Watzlaf, V. J. M., & Silverman, M. (1997). Development of a pilot quality assessment tool for long-term care facilities. *Topics in Health Information Management, 18*(1), 23–31.

108 Patyk, M., Gaynor, S., & Verdin, J. (2000). Patient education resource assessment: Project management. *Journal of Nursing Care Quality, 14*(2), 14–20.

47 Pearson, J. L., Lee, J. L., Chang, B. L., Elliott, M., Kahn, K. L., & Rubenstein, L. V. (2000). Structured implicit review: A new method for monitoring nursing care quality. *Medical Care, 38*(11), 1074–1091.

63 Peruzzi, M., Ringer, D., & Tassey, K. (1995). A community hospital redesigns care *Nursing Administration Quarterly, 20*(1), 24–46.

82 Philbin, E. F., Rogers, V. A,. Sheesley, K. A., Lynch, L. J. , Andreou, C., & Rocco, T. A., Jr. (1997). The relationship between hospital length of stay and rate of death in heart failure. *Heart & Lung: Journal of Acute & Critical Care, 26*(3),177–186.

82 Philbin, E.F., Lynch, L.J., Rocco, T.A., Lindenmuth, N.W., Ulrich, K., McCall, M., Jenkins, P., & Roerden, J. B. (1996). Does QI work? The management to improve survival in congestive heart failure (MISCHF) study. *Journal on Quality Improvement, 22*(11), 721–733.

120 Phillips, C. D., Spry, K. M., Sloane, P. D., & Hawes, C. (2000). Use of physical restraints and psychotropic medications in Alzheimer special care units in nursing homes. *American Journal of Public Health, 90*(1), 92–96.

129 Phillips, C. D., Zimmerman, D., Bernabei, R., & Jonsson, P. V. (1997). Using the Resident Assessment Instrument for quality enhancement in nursing homes. *Age & Ageing, 26*(Suppl 2), 77–81.

74 Phillips, K. F., & Crain, H. C. (1998). Effectiveness of a pneumonia clinical pathway: Quality and financial outcomes. *Outcomes Management for Nursing Practice, 2*(1), 16–23.

29 Phillips, L. R., Morrison, E., Steffl, B., Chae, Y. M., Cromwell, S. L., & Russell, C. K. (1995). Effects of the situational context and interactional process on the quality of family caregiving. *Research in Nursing & Health, 18*(3), 205–216.

31 Piercy, K. W., & Woolley, D. N. (1999). Negotiating worker-client relationships: A necessary step to providing quality home health care. *Home Health Care Services Quarterly, 18*(1),1–24.

124 Porell, F., & Caro, F. G. (1998). Facility-level outcome performance measures for nursing homes. *Gerontologist, 38*(6), 665–683.

R

98 Radwin, L. (2000). Oncology patients' perceptions of quality nursing care. *Research in Nursing & Health, 23*(3), 179–190.

98   Radwin, L., & Alster, K. (1999). Outcomes of perceived quality nursing care reported by oncology patients. *Scholarly Inquiry for Nursing Practice, 13*(4), 327–343, 345–347.

83   Rantz, M., Davis, N. K., & Tapp, R. A. (1995). Assessing elderly acute care services: Improving quality amid chaos. *Journal of Nursing Care Quality, 9*(3), 1–9.

130   Rantz, M. J., Mehr, D. R., Conn, V. S., Hicks, L. L., Porter, R., Madsen, R. W., Petroski, G. F., & Maas, M. (1996). Assessing quality of nursing home care: The foundation for improving resident outcomes. *Journal of Nursing Care Quality, 10*(4), 1–9.

125   Rantz, M. J., Mehr, D. R., Petroski, G. F., Madsen, R. W., Popejoy, L. L., Hicks, L. L., Conn, V. S., Grando, V. T., Wipke-Tevis, D. D., Bostick, J., Porter, R., Zwygart-Stauffacher, M., & Maas, M.(2000). Initial field testing of an instrument to measure: Observable indicators of nursing home care quality. *Journal of Nursing Care Quality, 14*(3), 1–12.

124   Rantz, M. J., Mehr, D. R., Popejoy, L., Zwygart-Stauffacher, M., Hicks, L. L., Grando, V., Conn, C. S., Porter, R., Scott, J., & Maas, M. (1998). Nursing home care quality: A multidimensional theoretical model. *Journal of Nursing Care Quality, 12*(3), 30–46, 69–70.

130   Rantz, M. J., Popejoy, L., Mehr, D. R, Zwygart-Stauffacher, M., Hicks, LL., Grando, V., Conn, V. S., Porter, R., Scott, J., & Maas, M. (1997). Verifying nursing home care quality using Minimum Data Set quality indicators and other quality measures. *Journal of Nursing Care Quality, 12*(2), 54–62.

125   Rantz, M. J., Zwygart-Stauffacher, M., Popejoy, L., Grando, V. T., Mehr, D. R., Hicks, L. L., Conn, V. S., Wipke-Tevis, D., Porter, R., Bostick, J., & Maas, M. (1999). Nursing home care quality: A multidimensional theoretical model integrating the views of consumers and providers. *Journal of Nursing Care Quality, 14*(1), 16–37, 85–87.

131   Rantz, M. J, Petroski, G. F., Madsen, R. W., Scott, J., Mehr, D. R., Popejoy, L., Hicks, L. L., Porter, R., Zwygart-Stauffacher, M., & Grando, V. T. (1997). Setting thresholds for MDS quality indicators for nursing home quality improvement reports. *Journal of Quality Improvement, 23*(11), 602–611.

131   Rantz, M. J., Petroski, G. F., Madsen, R. W., Mehr, D. R., Popejoy, L., Hicks, L. L., Porter, R., Zwygart-Stauffacher, M., & Grando, V. (2000). Setting thresholds for quality indicators derived from MDS data for nursing home quality improvement reports: An update. *Journal on Quality Improvement, 26*(2), 101–110.

103   Raper, J. L. (1996). A cognitive approach to patient satisfaction with emergency department nursing care. *Journal of Nursing Care Quality, 10*(4), 48–58.

104   Raper, J., Davis, B. A., & Scott, L. (1999). Patient satisfaction with emergency department triage nursing care: A multicenter study. *Journal of Nursing Care Quality, 13*(6), 11–24.

44   Redmond, G., & Sorrell, J. (1999). Studying patient satisfaction: Patient voices of quality. *Outcomes Management for Nursing Practice, 3*(2), 667–72.

44   Reed, L. Blegen, M. A., & Goode, C. S. (1998). Adverse patient occurrences as a measure of nursing care quality. *Journal of Nursing Administration, 28*(5), 62–69.

31   Riccio, P. A. (2000). Quality evaluation of home nursing care: Perceptions of patients, physicians, and nurses. *Nursing Administration Quarterly, 24*(3), 43–52.

98   Richmond, I., & Roberson, E. (1995). The customer is always right: Patients' perceptions of psychiatric nursing actions. *Journal of Nursing Care Quality, 9*(2), 36–43.

83   Riegel, B., Gates, D. M., Gocka, I., Medina, L., Odell, C., Rich, M., & Finken, J. S. (1996). Effectiveness of a program of early hospital discharge of cardiac surgery patients

[corrected] [published erratum appears in *J Cardiovasc Nurs* 1997 Apr; 11(3), viii]. *Journal of Cardiovascular Nursing, 11*(1), 63–75.

83 Roman, S., Linekin, P., & Stagnaro-Green, A. (1995). An inpatient diabetes QI program. *The Joint Commission Journal on Quality Improvement, 21*(12), 693–699.

99 Rosenfeld, P., Duthie, E., Bier, J., Bowar-Ferres, S., Fulmer, T,. Iervolino, L., McClure, M. L., McGivern, D. O., & Roncoli, M. (2000). Engaging staff nurses in evidence-based research to identify nursing practice problems and solutions. *Applied Nursing Research, 13*(4), 197–203.

84 Rumble, S. J., Jernigan, M. H., & Rudisill, P. T. (1996). Determining the effectiveness of critical pathways for coronary bypass graft patients: Retrospective comparison of readmission rates. *Journal of Nursing Care Quality, 11*(2), 34–40.

S

99 Sales, A., Lurie, N., Moscovice, I., & Goes, J. (1995). Is quality in the eye of the beholder? *The Joint Commission Journal on Quality Improvement, 21*(5), 219–225.

59 Sayers, M., Marando, R., Fisher, S., Aquila, A., Morrison, B., & Dailey, T. (2000). No need for pain. *Journal for Healthcare Quality, 22*(3), 10–14.

104 Schaffer, P., Vaughn, G., Kenner, C., Donohue, F., & Longo, A. (2000). Revision of a parent satisfaction survey based on the parent perspective. *Journal of Pediatric Nursing: Nursing Care of Children & Families, 15*(6), 373–377.

47 Schell, J. A., Bynum, C. G., Lynan, K. L., & Shaul, B. (2000). Survival analysis in quality improvement: The diabetic kidney disease project extrapolation group estimates. *Journal for Healthcare Quality, 22*(4), 37–44

146 Scherb, C. A., Rapp, C. G., Johnson, M., & Maas, M. (1998). The Nursing Outcomes Classification: Validation by rehabilitation nurses. *Rehabilitation Nursing, 23*(4), 174–178, 191.

142 Schifalacqua, M., Hook, M., O'Hearn, P., & Schmidt, M. (2000). Coordinating the care of the chronically ill in a world of managed care. *Nursing Administration Quarterly, 24*(3), 12–20.

128 Schirm, V., Albanese, T., & Garland, T. N. (1999). Understanding nursing home quality of care: Incorporating caregivers' perceptions through structure, process, and outcome. *Quality Management in Health Care, 8*(1), 55–63.

127 Schirm, V., Albanese, T., Garland, T. N., Gipson, G., & Blackmon, D. J. (2000). Caregiving in nursing homes: Views of licensed nurses and nursing assistants. *Clinical Nursing Research, 9*(3), 280–297.

32 Schlenker, R. E., Hittle, D. F., & Arnold, A. G. (1995). Home health agency quality: Medicare certification findings compared to patient outcomes. *Home Health Care Services Quarterly, 15*(4), 97–115.

48 Schwab, R. A., DelSorbo, S. M., Cunningham, M. R., Craven, K., & Watson, W. A. (1999). Using statistical process control to demonstrate the effect of operational interventions on quality indicators in the emergency department. *Journal for Healthcare Quality, 21*(4), 38–41.

84 Shedd, P. P., Kobokovich, L. J., & Slattery, J. S. (1995). Confused patients in the acute care setting: Prevalence, interventions, and outcomes. *Journal of Gerontological Nursing, 21*(4), 5–12.

120 Sheppard, C. M., & Brenner, P. S. (2000). The effects of bathing and skin care prac-

tices on skin quality and satisfaction with an innovative product. *Journal of Gerontological Nursing, 26*(10), 36–45.

59 Sherwood, G., Adams-McNeill, J., Starck, P. L., Nieto, B., & Thompson, C. J. (2000). Qualitative assessment of hospitalized patients' satisfaction with pain management. *Research in Nursing & Health, 23*(6), 486–495.

141 Shindul-Rothschild, J., Berry, D., & Long-Middleton, E. (1997). Where have all the nurses gone? Final results of AJN's patient care survey. *MCN, American Journal of Maternal Child Nursing, 22*(1), 33–47.

104 Silberzweig, J., & Giguere, B. (1996). Redesign for patient satisfaction. *Journal of Nursing Care Quality, 11*(2), 25–33.

89 Siminoff, L. A., Erlen, J. A., & Sereika, S. (1998). Do nurses avoid AIDS patients? Avoidance behaviors and the quality of care of hospitalized AIDS patients. *AIDS Care, 10*(2), 147–163.

121 Simmons, S. F., & Schnelle, J. F. (1999). Strategies to measure nursing home residents' satisfaction and preferences related to incontinence and mobility care: Implications for evaluating intervention effects. *Gerontologist, 39*(3), 345–355.

75 Simonds, D. N., Horan, T. C., Kelley R., & Jarvis, W. R. (1997). Detecting pediatric nosocomial infections: How do infection control and quality assurance personnel compare? *American Journal of Infection Control, 25*(3), 202–208.

128 Singh, D. A., Amidon, R. L., Shi, L., & Samuels, M. E. (1996). Predictors of quality of care in nursing facilities. *Journal of Long Term Care Administration, 24*(3), 22–26.

139 Sloss, E. M., Solomon, D. H., Shekelle, P. G., Young, R. T., Saliba, D., MacLean, C. H., Rubenstein, L. Z., Schnelle, J. F., Kamberg, C. J., & Wenger, N. S. (2000). Selecting target conditions for quality of care improvement in vulnerable older adults. *Journal of the American Geriatrics Society, 48*(4), 363–369.

67 Sochalski, J., Estabrooks, C. A., & Humphrey, C. K. (1999). Nurse staffing and patient outcomes: Evolution of an international study. *Canadian Journal of Nursing Research, 31*(3), 69–88.

134 Specht, J. P., Kelley, L. S., Manion, P., Maas, M. L., Reed, D., & Rantz, M. R. (2000). Who's the boss? Family/staff partnership in care of persons with dementia. *Nursing Administration Quarterly, 24*(3), 64–75.

60 Starck, P. L., Adams, J., Sherwood, G., & Thompson, C. (1997). Development of a pain management report card for an acute care setting. *Advanced Practice Nursing Quarterly, 3*(2), 57–63.

132 Steffen, T. M., & Nystrom, P. C. (1997). Validation of a measure of family members' perceptions of service quality in nursing homes. *Journal of Rehabilitation Outcomes Measurement, 1*(4), 1–9.

55 Stetler, C. B., Morsi, D., & Burns, M. (2000). Physical and emotional patient safety: A different look at nursing-sensitive outcomes. *Outcomes Management for Nursing Practice, 4*(4), 159–166.

121 Stevenson, K. B. (1999). Regional data set of infection rates for long-term care facilities: Description of a valuable benchmarking tool. *American Journal of Infection Control, 27*(1), 20–26.

60 Stratton, L. (1999). Evaluating the effectiveness of a hospital's pain management program. *Journal of Nursing Care Quality, 13*(4), 8–18.

67 Strzalka, A., & Havens, D. S. (1996). Nursing care quality: Comparison of unit-hired, hospital float pool, and agency nurses. *Journal of Nursing Care Quality, 10*(4), 59–65.

56   Swauger, K. C., & Tomlin, C. C. (2000). Moving toward restraint-free patient care. *Journal of Nursing Administration, 30*(6), 325–329.

T

52   Thompson, D. G., & Maringer, M. (1995). Using case management to improve care delivery in the NICU. *MCN, American Journal of Maternal Child Nursing, 20*(5), 257–260.

135 Tolle, S. W., Tilden, V. P., Nelson, C. A., Dunn, & P. M. (1998). A prospective study of the efficacy of the physician order form for life-sustaining treatment. *Journal of the American Geriatrics Society, 46*(9), 1097–1102.

U

72   Urden, L. D. (1996). Development of a nurse executive decision support database: A model for outcomes evaluation. *Journal of Nursing Administration, 26*(10), 15–20.

V

21   Van Acker, B., McIntosh, G., & Gudes, M. (1998). Continuous quality improvement techniques enhance HMO members' immunization rates. *Journal for Healthcare Quality, 20*(2), 36–41.

92   Van Ess Coeling, H., & Cukr, P. L. (2000). Communication styles that promote perceptions of collaboration, quality, and nurse satisfaction. *Aspens Advisor for Nurse Executives, 15*(11), 1–12.

122 Van Ort, S., & Phillips, L. R. (1995). Nursing interventions to promote functional feeding. *Journal of Gerontological Nursing, 21*(10), 7–14.

105 VanderVeen, L., & Ritz, M. (1996). Customer satisfaction: A practical approach for hospitals. *Journal for Healthcare Quality, 18*(2), 10–15.

W

132 Wakefield B., Buckwalter, K. C., & Collins, C. E. (1997). Assessing family satisfaction with care for persons with dementia. *Balance, 1*(1), 16–7, 40–42.

45   Wakefield, D. S., Hendryx , M. S., Uden-Holman, T., Couch, R., & Helms, C. M. (1996). Comparing providers' performance: Problems in making the "report card" analogy fit. *Journal for Healthcare Quality: Promoting Excellence in Healthcare, 18*(6), 4–10.

22   Walker, P. H., Baker, J. J., & Chiverton, P. (1998). Costs of interdisciplinary practice in a school-based health center. *Outcomes Management for Nursing Practice, 2*(1), 37–44.

84   Wammack, L., & Mabrey, J. D. (1998). Outcomes assessment of total hip and total knee arthroplasty: Critical pathways, variance analysis, and continuous quality improvement. *Clinical Nurse Specialist, 12*(3), 122–131.

53   Waters, J. B., Wolff, R. S., Blansfield, J., LaMorte, W.W., Millham, F. H., & Hirsch, E. F. (1999). Development and implementation of clinical pathways for the management of four trauma diagnoses. *Journal for Healthcare Quality, 21*(3), 4–11.

133 Watson, C. J., Mobarak, A. M., & Stimson, K. (1999). A collaborative effort to establish a long-term care benchmark process. *Journal for Healthcare Quality, 21*(2), 19–23.

111 Weaver, F. M., Conrad, K. J., Guihan ,M., Byck, G. R., Manheim, L. M., & Hughes, S.L. (1996). Evaluation of a prospective payment system for VA contract nursing homes. *Evaluation & the Health Professions, 19*(4), 423–442.

85   Whitcomb, R., & Aleman, D. (1995). Achieving excellence in thrombolytic therapy. *Journal for Healthcare Quality, 17*(3), 23–25, 38.

99   Williams, S. A. (1998). Quality and care: Patients' perceptions. *Journal of Nursing Care Quality, 12*(6), 18–25, 70–72.

105 Williams, S. A. (1997). The relationship of patients' perceptions of holistic nurse caring to satisfaction with nursing care. *Journal of Nursing Care Quality, 11*(5),15–29.

89   Wise, L. C., Mersch, J., Racioppi, J., Crosier, J., & Thompson, C. (2000). Evaluating the reliability and utility of cumulative intake and output. *Journal of Nursing Care Quality, 14*(3), 37–42.

105 Wolf, Z. R., Colahan, M., Costello, A. , Warwick, F., Ambrose, M. S., & Giardino, E. R. (1998). Research utilization. Relationship between nurse caring and patient satisfaction. *MEDSURG Nursing, 7*(2), 99–105.

Y

85   York, R., Brown, L. P., Samuels, P., Finkler, S. A., Jacobsen, B., Persely, C. A., Swank, A., & Robbins, D. (1997). A randomized trial of early discharge and nurse specialist transitional follow-up care of high-risk childbearing women. *Nursing Research, 46*(5), 254–261.

100 Young, W. B., Minnick, A. F., & Marcantonio, R. (1996). How wide is the gap in defining quality care? Comparison of patient and nurse perceptions of important aspects of patient care. *Journal of Nursing Administration, 26*(5), 15–20.

Z

56   Zollo, M. B., Gostisha, M .L., Berens, R .J., Schmidt, J. E., & Weigle, C. G. M. (1996). Altered skin integrity in children admitted to a pediatric intensive care unit. *Journal of Nursing Care Quality, 11*(2), 62–67.

141 Zwygart-Stauffacher, M., Lindquist, R., Savik, K. (2000). Development of health care delivery systems that are sensitive to the needs of stroke survivors and their caregivers. *Nursing Administration Quarterly, 24*(3), 33–42.

Index

Psychiatric and psychosocial topics
adult patients, 50–51, 86, 89, 92, 98–99
geriatric patients, 27, 77, 84, 103, 118, 119, 120, 122, 123, 127–28, 132–33, 134, 139
See also Dementia/confusion; Depression

Q

Quality (discussed), 1–3
Quality improvement, 3, 7
in ambulatory care, 11–13
cross-setting, 137–39
home health, 26–29
hospital care (VA), 37, 110–11
Quality indicators, 38
Quality measurement, 3, 6–7
long term care, 122–26
methods (hospitals), 46–49
nurse-sensitive outcomes and, 3, 6*t*, 145
Quality outcomes
in ambulatory care, 10–11
classification, 145
community health care, 20–22
home health care, 26–29
hospital-based care, 40–46
Quality perceptions, 94–101

S

Satisfaction with care. *See* Patient satisfaction
School health care, 19
Skin integrity topics
in geriatrics, 120–21

in pediatrics, 57–58
Staff and staffing issues
hospital-based, 38, 65–69, 90–94
long-term care, 126–28
staff perceptions, 29–31, 38
Standardized nursing language, 7
Standards, 2
Stroke topics, 78, 140, 141
Surgery topics 59, 70, 76, 77, 80, 82, 84, 95
post-op, 76, 106, 138
transplant and replacement, 78–79

T

Terminology (discussed), 1–3
THR/TKR (total hip replacement/total knee replacement), 78, 84–85
Transplant and replacement surgery, 78–79
Trauma, emergency room situations 48, 53, 104

V

Vascular/venous access topics, 46, 86–87, 88–89, 119
Veterans Affairs (VA) hospital care, 6*t*, 109
clinical issues, 109–10
quality improvement, 110–11

W

Weight and nutrition issues, 35, 117, 118, 122, 139
Women's health topics, viii*t*
Work environment (hospitals), 90–94